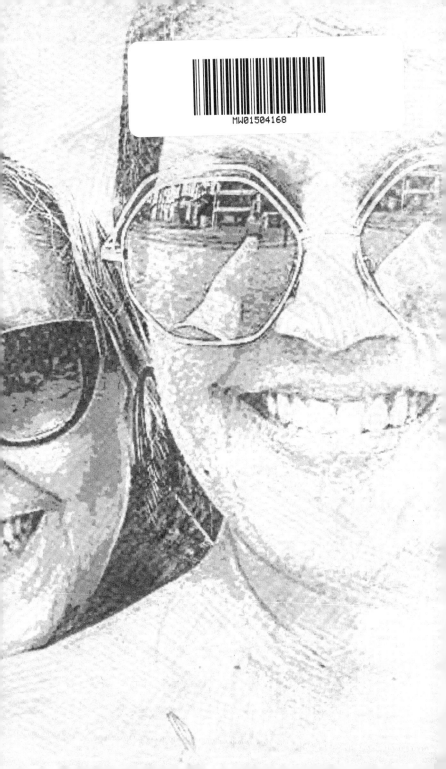

Handle
With Care
Your Breast Cancer Support Group in a Book

ISBN: 9798657699821
ISBN-13: 979-8657699821

Cover design and interior layout, Steven Lesh

The CARE Project, Inc., First edition (August 1st, 2020)

HWC Book Print 2e - FINAL

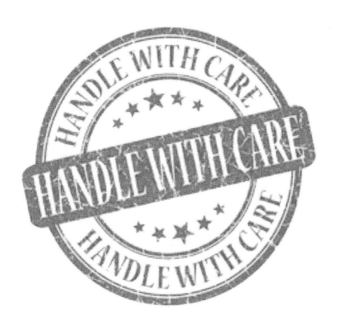

This book is dedicated to all of the breast cancer patients who have crossed the finish line of life before us. We know that in some way their breast cancer experience helped us through ours.

When a breast cancer patient dies, we often hear the phrase, "Lost their battle," but we choose to believe they earned their wings to be free from disease and suffering. Their mission was accomplished on Earth. Somewhere, they are dancing in the sky and sprinkling bravery, positivity, and pixie dust all over us as we walk the path of cancer treatment and recovery.

Special angels we miss dearly: Nancy Belk, Shannon K. Brown, Angelica Cardenas, Nashaka Foster, Elsa Garza, Adrienne Gracia, Robert Holden, Jennifer Lake, Ivette Martinez, Mike Phillips, Monica Price.

> "The highest form of wisdom is kindness."
> ~ The Talmud

Contents

Forward • Reading Others' Stories • Telling Our Own Stories • So What Have We Learned about Power and Inspiration?

85 / **What Surprised Us**

You Think You Know People • Accepting Help from Others • Perspective • Harsh Financial Reality • Scanxiety is Real • There is So Much to Learn • Learning the Hard Way • If Someone Offers You Help, Take It • A Newer You • Our Circle • Outlook • So What We Have Learned about What Surprised Us?

93 / **What We Don't Want to Hear**

Free Tummy Tuck! • Don't Say This • Or This • Unsolicited Opinions • Advice not Needed! • Call Me! • Free Boobs! Get Them Here! • Blanket Generalizations • What? No Reconstruction? Gasp! • Leave the Conspiracy Theories at Home, Please • But Your Hair! • Sometimes We're not Strong, and that's Okay • So What Do We Want to Hear?

103 / **Support Groups**

Definitely not a Bad Lifetime Movie • Surrogate Family • Lifelong Friends • The Right Fit for You • They Really Get Me! • There Wasn't One for Me, So I Created One • It's Funny How One Thing Leads to Another • Not All Rainbows and Sunshine (things get real) • You are not Alone • You do You • Voices of Experience, Mentors • Helped Mourn My Loss • There is a Group for Everyone • So What Have We Learned about Support Groups?

An Introduction

After I wrote about my own life-changing experiences with breast cancer back in 2013, I began hearing from others whose lives had also been impacted—not just by breast cancer, but by the "Big C" in general. The experience transforms us, changing our outlook on life, forcing us to pause and do some major stock-taking. Of everything. We ask ourselves big questions like: Where do we want to take this one extraordinary life? How do we want to use our finite time? What will our legacy be?

Not insignificant, these Big Life Things.

The more people I connected with, whether chatting over emails, finding each other online, or meeting in real life, the more I realized: While some cancer truths are universal, such as the punch-to-the-gut shock that comes from hearing the words, "You have cancer," I soon learned each of us has our own unique perspective and story to share. We each have a few things we had to learn the hard way, the "If only I had known in the beginning" things.

In 2016, I met Carrie Madrid, co-founder of The CARE Project, Inc., her local support organization she built from the ground up with the help and support of her close friend Christina Gonzalez. The CARE Project, Inc. is the product of what Carrie calls her "Big, Bright Idea" to help fill the emotional void faced by those recently diagnosed, especially after their initial web of family and friend support has faded. After Carrie's diagnosis of Stage III invasive ductal carcinoma in 2012, several surgeries, a battle with a deadly staph infection, even more surgeries, and a lengthy recovery process, she became determined to create something more than simply an emotional support group. Her Big Bright Idea: Build a social club where breast cancer patients feel comfortable enough to hang out, let their hair (and wigs) down, show their scars, cry their tears, and laugh until they're doubled over. In short, a group where everyone gets it.

Carrie is an example of being the change we want to see in the world, and this book, like The CARE Project, Inc., is the product of our collective Hive Mind: Women and men in the breast cancer community sharing unique perspectives on everything from treatment to epiphanies, life moments, funny stories, and poignant truths. Things we wish we knew in the beginning of our treatment as well as things we'd like friends and those playing support roles to know. Think of this as your support group in a book. Real talk about our fears, the numbness, the shock, and what helped get us through.

[*All proceeds from the sales of this book benefit The CARE Project, Inc., in furtherance of their mission to provide emotional and financial support to the newly diagnosed as well as long-term wellness for those in treatment, survivors, and thrivers.*]

Our wish is that every person who reads Handle With CARE will find comfort and know that you are not alone. We are a hive, and you are part of us now. ~

Margaret Lesh, *author of Let Me Get This Off My Chest*
Carrie Madrid, *Co-Founder of The CARE Project, Inc.*

Handle With Care

small **our gang...**

Meet the Hive:

- Carrie Madrid
- Lavetta Ross
- T.H. Hernandez
- Ayanna Clark
- Diana Jaurigue
- Kayte Faulconer

- Christina Villanueva
- S.L. Huang
- Bret Miller
- Kay Hsu
- Gina Negrete Fitzsimmons
- Margaret Lesh

First, The Inspiration Behind Carrie's Motto...

- *"Laughter & Lip Gloss"* -

Carrie • The day I was diagnosed, I left the surgeon's office with my best friend, and she said to me, "Well, now what are we going to do?"

I said, "We're going to the mall, and we're buying lip gloss."

"We're doing WHAT?"

"We're going to go to Nordstrom, and we're going to buy the expensive lip gloss." I meant the kind that a single mom never buys, because you just don't spend money on that kind of stuff. There was this brand that I had my eye on but never felt like I could justify the expense—not with kids at home to take care of.

We went to the mall, and I bought two of the most expensive tubes of lip gloss that I could find. I decided right then: My motto through this is going to be "Laughter and Lip Gloss," because I can either laugh or I can cry, and I'm going to choose to laugh my way through while I can. And, if nothing else, when I lose my eyelashes, eyebrows, and all the rest, I can always keep my lip gloss on.

I also promised her to keep my toenails polished.

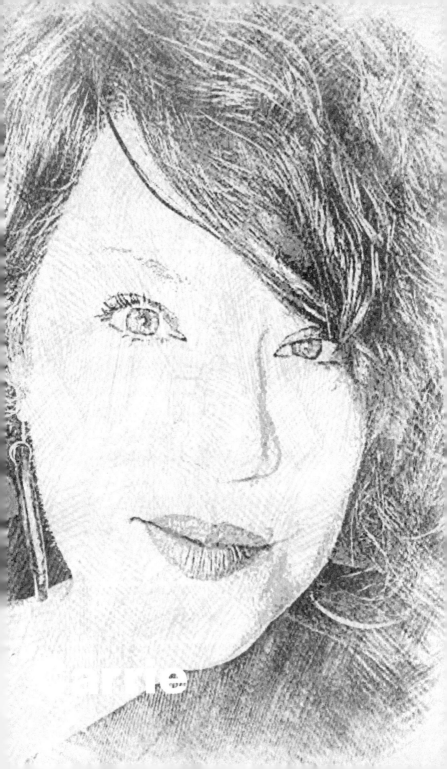

Diagnosis

A diagnosis of breast cancer means suddenly being on the receiving end of a dizzying amount of information. In a state of numbed shock, we are asked to make huge choices such as what type of live-saving surgery we will undergo—lumpectomy? mastectomy? one breast? both?—to what oncologist and/or surgeon we will choose; whether we will undergo chemotherapy and/or radiation; whether we will take medication to suppress our hormones, placing us into early menopause; whether we will undergo genetic testing to determine if other family members are at risk, and so on. We soon find ourselves being carried along in a series of appointments, procedures, poking, prodding, and endless waiting. There is a massive amount of data to process all at once.

The Hive discusses their own diagnoses—what it felt like, and how we got through it—with a few words of wisdom:

- *a word of advice* -

Carrie • I think you really need to take it all in and really kind of sit with the information for a little bit before you start—I don't want to say making decisions, that's obvious, but I think we all go into that panic mode, and I think we really need to sit and look at it as reflectively as we can. Have maybe one or two people that aren't related to you, maybe friends that are calm, pretty even-keeled, that you can go to that will help you talk through it because when you're dealing with your family, they're probably all emotional too.

If you can find that one calming friend—it might not even be someone that you're super close with but that you're comfortable with—to kind of talk things through with, that helps. I did have a couple friends like that. They weren't freaking out like family were, and that helped me.

- *bring someone to take notes* -

Margaret • I was thirty-four with no family history of breast cancer when I received my diagnosis of Stage I invasive ductal carcinoma. In those first few days (weeks) operating on shellshocked auto-pilot mode, what helped was having someone with me during my appointments to act as a second set of ears to help process the incoming flood of information. My suggestion to anyone, especially in the beginning, is to have a family member or friend accompany you to your doctors' appointments to take notes and be that second set of eyes and ears.

- *the waiting is the hardest part* -

T.H. • I was diagnosed in January of 2016, just two days after my brother-in-law lost a very short battle with pancreatic cancer. My children, all young teens at the time, watched their uncle succumb to a disease that robbed him of everything that made him who he was in their eyes. To say that breaking the news to them was my biggest anxiety would be a gross understatement. The only thing worse than telling my kids was telling my parents. Luckily, my sister took that bullet for me.

From the minute I made an appointment with my OB/GYN

Handle With Care

because my nipple looked funny until I received my diagnosis six long weeks later, I was an absolute wreck. I couldn't sleep, barely ate, and mostly went through the motions of life. But the very second my doctor looked me in the eye and said I had breast cancer, the fog lifted. The veil of uncertainty was gone and I had my answer. I didn't know what was going to happen next, but at least I knew something.

It's true what Tom Petty said, the waiting really is the hardest part.

- *swimming with sharks* -

S.L. • The moment of diagnosis is sharp, acute, a surrealism that sticks in memory. Like plunging into the deep end of a pool, only with sharks, and the suffocating certainty I'm never going to come back up. I've had a diagnosis moment twice, and I remember both like those instants were carved into my brain with knives. But the sharpness will abate. It'll be replaced with a longer, duller ache of doctors, needles, uncertainty, the monotony of medical torture one day after the next. The nightmare will become a new normal. It's both easier and harder than going underwater that first time— the good thing about plunging is that it's over quickly, even as it leaves the rest.

- *my diagnosis* -

Christina • I was diagnosed the first time in 1997 at the age of twenty-two. The second time around, it came back at age of forty-five in 2015 as triple negative.

Lavetta • I was originally diagnosed with Stage II breast cancer in March 2016. I found a lump in my breast, and I went to see my doctor. He started probing, you know, exploring with the tests and everything, and come to find out, it had originally said Stage II, but after the surgery and everything, I turned out to be Stage III, and it infiltrated five of my lymph nodes. They took out fifteen during the surgery, but it had gone into five.

Diana • My diagnosis was in December of 2013, and it was quite a surprise because it was right before Christmas, right before I was going on a trip to London and Spain. I couldn't go because of the fact that they found this mass behind the left nipple, and it was Stage III. So I had to cancel the trip, and it was overwhelming.

I was supposed to have gone in October for my mammogram —my mammograms are always in October, because of Breast Cancer Awareness Month—but I had put it off until right before Thanksgiving. I was going to put it off again, because I was going to wait until I returned from my trip to do it. Luckily, something told me: Go. Just go.

I had no symptoms whatsoever. I didn't have any swelling; I didn't have any pain; I didn't feel anything different.

I went for my mammogram the week before Thanksgiving, and the Monday after Thanksgiving is when they said that it was abnormal but not to worry, these things happen; come back and have an ultrasound. I had my ultrasound, and they immediately said, "You need to come in and have a biopsy." The week before Christmas is when it came back that it was definitely positive. It was just very, very scary, because no one had had breast cancer in my family. It was quite a shock.

- *I am a survivor* -

Kayte • I was diagnosed with Stage IIB invasive ductal carcinoma at thirty-three years old, estrogen and progestin positive, HER2 negative. I opted for a bilateral mastectomy and had it done only eight days after being diagnosed. It was a definite whirlwind.

Still feels funny to say it, sometimes. Very surreal. I am a cancer survivor.

- *how did you handle it?* -

Carrie • When I was first diagnosed, people would later ask me, "How did you handle it?" The first thing that comes to mind is when I was in the surgeon's office, and he told me the results, I was really at peace with it. What I mean by that is I wasn't okay with it, but I wasn't shocked, and I wasn't scared to death in that moment. Okay, I was probably in shock a little bit—technically in shock a little bit—but I remember my friend saying to me, "How can you be so calm?"

I said, "You know what? I have two daughters at home, and I have thirty-two basketball daughters who all call me 'Mom,' and some day one out of eight of them could be diagnosed, and they're going to always be able to look back and remember how I handled it. So maybe, in part, this is for them."

At that point, I had this peace. I was still afraid, obviously, of what was to come in terms of treatment, but I knew that I was going to live through it. I think those girls, knowing that they were watching me, really kept me as calm as I could be ninety-eight percent of the time.

- *Sarah's story, and mine* -

Gina • My story doesn't start with my diagnosis, it starts with my friend Sarah's. She was breastfeeding her one year old and found a lump that would turn out to be triple negative breast cancer. She had a double mastectomy, started treatment, and they thought that she was good to go, but within six months, it had spread.

We were family acquaintances, but as soon as she was diagnosed, something inside of me told me that I wanted to be there for her and be her support group. We started communicating and talking via social media a little more, and Sarah also shared her story publicly via social media. She wound up having thousands of followers where she shared about every office visit, what type of chemo, radiation, the surgeries—all that she endured.

We formed a bond, and I was there through everything. A year and a half later, in 2017, I'm in my surgeon's office, and she's telling me that I have Stage I triple negative breast cancer. So for me, the Lord has taken care of me through Sarah's fight. Sarah taught me everything that I ever needed to know about cancer. She taught me what it looked like; what a fighter looked like. She taught me what to expect; she taught me about the treatment.

She taught me to be my own advocate.

- *my concerns were passed off* -

Ayanna • I was diagnosed in March of 2017 with triple negative breast cancer, Stage II or III. But I had several symptoms before that including breast pain, an inverted nipple, nipple discharge,

Handle With Care

and a change in breast appearance.

After numerous appointments—including one with a female breast surgeon—I was told: "Breast cancer doesn't hurt"; "Lots of women have breast pain"; and to stop drinking caffeine. That was in the last months of 2016.

I also had a mammogram in late 2016 on my right breast only, because at the time the doctor was only able to get the discharge from that breast—even when I told her the pain and discharge were occurring in both.

I should have fought for it—for myself—but I didn't.

The mammogram came back clean, so I went on with living, figuring I was a true hypochondriac, only to find a large lump in my left breast in January 2017. There were two lumps in my left breast and cancer was detected in my lymph nodes. I chose to have a double mastectomy.

If I can emphasize one thing, it's: Trust your body; trust yourself. Be your own advocate and get a second or even third opinion.

- *annual screenings* -

Diana • I can't stress enough the importance of annual mammograms. I've met so many women who are in their early thirties—a couple even in their late twenties—that are being diagnosed with breast cancer. They're told they don't need their mammograms unless they're in their forties.

If you feel anything, or if it runs in your family, you need to go.

What I have found from this whole experience is that we

have to be our own advocates. If your doctor says, "No, you're too young for that," you have to say, "I have to have it done. I don't want to wait until I'm forty."

That's what I would stress to whoever is reading this: You have to be your own advocate. You have to get educated on what's going on. Because we know how our bodies respond and how they deal with certain things, and no one else knows that.

Hive Diagnosis Tips:

• If you are able to take someone with you to appointments, do.

• As much as possible, take it one day, one appointment, at a time.

• Try not to do too much time traveling to every "what-if" scenario your mind can torment you with.

• Before you know it, you will shift from numbed shock to a more functional, auto-pilot new normal, and that's okay.

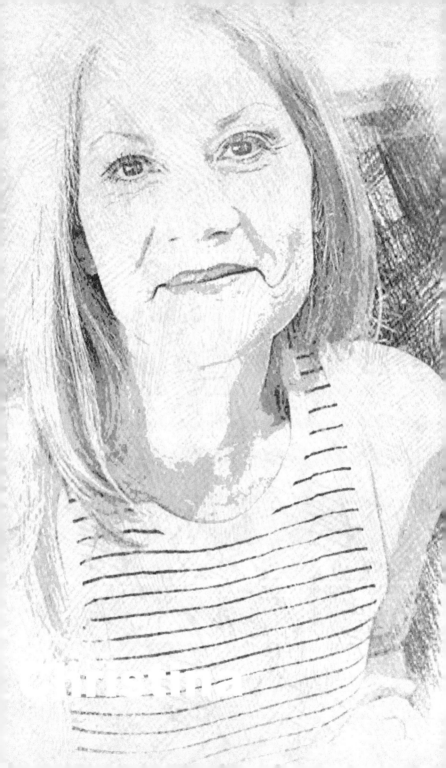

Chemotherapy

The word "chemotherapy" is enough to strike fear into our hearts; we've all heard about the terrible things that people go through during the process. Much of our fear, though, is from the unknowns and the "what-ifs."

"Will I get sick every time?

"Can I work during treatments?"

"Will I lose my hair?"

One sure thing is that no two people will have the exact chemo experience. Just as we each have our own unique stories, so will be our individual response to chemotherapy as well as the regimen. We might receive infusions weekly, biweekly, or once a month. Our chemo may also come in the form of a medication taken daily for five years, ten years, or more.

One general, loose guideline to keep in mind: One step, one infusion, one day at a time.

The Hive weighs in on chemo:

- *don't go it alone, if you can help it* -

Carrie • Because I had such a harsh regimen, knowing what I know now, I would suggest that you have at least one person go with you to every treatment. And not just go with you, but to stay with you that night, because I was Ms. Badass, "Oh, just take me there and get me home, I'll be fine." But truly, those were the scary nights for me, right after treatment.

- *counting down* -

Kayte • I had a combination of Taxotere and Cytoxan every three weeks and had a total of six sessions. The side effects were pretty minimal at first but definitely grew over time. The last two sessions I felt the most and was the most miserable. I had a countdown app going—for my last chemo—and would post updates on Facebook so that all of my family and friends could count down with me.

- *each of us is different* -

Christina • Everyone reacts differently to chemo, so don't listen to others, because it's never the same. I say to someone going through it to find a purpose to get through it just as I did. I found the purpose to live for my grand-baby the second time. The first time, my kids were little, and I wanted to live for them, especially with me being only twenty-two. I now see everything I endured and what came along with it such as love and support from people I didn't even know that now became my new family.

Handle With Care

- *chemo before surgery* -

Diana • A lot of women that I have been speaking to had surgery first, and then they had the chemo or then radiation, depending on what the diagnosis was. Mine, they decided to do chemo first, because it was more of a mass, and they wanted to see if they could shrink it and get clean borders. My chemo went from January through June, and it didn't do much at all. I mean, other than maintaining it. It maintained it, and it didn't spread any further.

- *on side effects* -

T.H. • While chemo is far from fun, it's nowhere near as awful as movies and TV shows portray it. At least not for most breast cancer patients. I had one of the strongest chemo cocktails out there, and I never vomited once. Not to say I didn't feel awful, because I did, but I was expecting it to be worse. Your doctor should send you home with anti-nausea meds as well as anti-diarrheals, so be sure to ask for them if they aren't offered.

Because my chemo was so powerful, I was a candidate for Neulasta to help me maintain some white blood cells. It works, but it can cause really awful bone pain. For whatever reason, taking a daily Claritin significantly reduces that pain, so ask your oncologist about it.

[*Neulasta (pegfilgrastim) is a man-made form of a protein that stimulates the growth of white blood cells in your body.*]

- *stay hydrated, people!* -

Carrie • I think physically, just drinking a ton of water is what got me through. I'm shocked by the amount of people I talk to who are going through chemo that don't drink water. How do you do that? So I say drink a ton of water for the physical aspect. And just as a backup, you should always have somebody around you, because you never know from one treatment to the next if you're going to have a reaction. My body reacted to each treatment differently.

Diana • I would get very, very nauseous, and I had to go back the next day for two to three hours of intravenous hydration in the chemo ward. That's the only thing that would help me, because if I would go to lie down, the room was spinning. Afterward, Pedialyte did help. I put it in the fridge and would have it ice cold, and I would take little sips on it after they would hydrate me. Also, wet towels on my forehead and around my neck. That's what would save me.

Ayanna • Chemo is rough, to put it lightly. After having my port inserted, I did my chemo treatment like everyone, but my port scar never healed, and it became infected. I was hospitalized for sepsis for almost a week. After that, I had a PICC placed, but that also didn't work out, and I had my last several chemo treatments intravenously in my arm. I did suffer from nausea and vomiting, but not as much as I expected.

[*Peripherally Inserted Central Catheter line.*]

Handle With Care

- *take the nausea meds!* -

Gina • I am allergic to everything—dogs, grass, food—so of course I was one of the small percentage of people allergic to chemo. I first got a pain in the pit of my stomach, which traveled up into my chest, and my face turned beet red. My sessions of Cisplatin (Red Devil) that were supposed to be four hours ended up being seven or eight to slow everything down. They gave me steroids in my I.V., and Benadryl—whatever I needed—to handle it.

My advice..? Take all the meds that they give you—ALL the medications—like the Zofran for nausea. A lot of people say, "I don't feel nauseous," but they don't because they're taking their meds. Then they stop taking it, and they start getting nauseous; now they're behind the medication. Try to stay ahead of it. Once you're behind, it's much harder to get back on track again. That's the one thing they did tell me. They're there for a reason— because other people have gone through it, and this is what they feel is most effective.

- *on fatigue* -

Lavetta • I actually worked while I was going through chemo. On the weeks that I had my treatment, I was off work a couple of days, and when I was in treatment—you know how you have those days where you're feeling okay, but then the next couple of days you feel like you've been hit by a truck? So tired. Those were the days I took off work. I just decided to work through it and continued to stay busy with work, and that's basically what I did.

Looking back on it, I wouldn't work. I would have taken the

whole year off. I worked three weeks before my surgery, and I should have been off sooner than that, because those three weeks, I realized I was really, really tired. Going into my surgery, I was really tired. So that's why I would advise: If you can take off work, take the time off.

- *on hair loss* -

T.H. • Besides losing my hair, which all women are understandably attached to, the hardest part of this leg of my journey was all the delays. My husband travels at least sixty percent of the time. He worked with his company to rearrange his schedule so he could attend all my chemo appointments with me. But my labs never cooperated. I have naturally low platelets that chemo took to dangerously low levels. What should have been chemo every three weeks turned into chemo every four weeks, dragging out this phase of treatment by six weeks and preventing my husband from attending more than two of those rounds with me. That was hard. I cried more about that than about my hair.

Christina • I had sixteen rounds of chemo with my recurrence but not the first time. When the doctor told me that I would be having sixteen rounds of chemo, it terrified me because of stories I'd heard of how harsh and painful it was. What terrified me the most was knowing I would be losing my hair. After the first round, I started to see chunks of hair coming out, and it made me feel like I was losing my womanhood.

Cancer had taken my breast already, on top of my hair as well. I know someone that hasn't gone through that will not understand, but I later learned that through the worst days of chemo, God did give me the strength to overcome it and make it through. Now I have a head full of hair again and don't think about my vanity anymore.

Ayanna • When I lost my hair, it was quite sad. I remember sitting at the table with my sister, who said something like, "Your hair is hanging on." I hadn't shared with anyone that I saw that it was falling out. I had natural hair, so the thickness concealed it. At the table I pulled a few strands out to show her. She left for an appointment, and when she returned, I had pretty much pulled all the hair out. (I have an extremely sad video of this.) My brother-in-law cut the rest off, and my mom cut hers off that same day in solidarity.

The worst part of it for me was when I lost my eyebrows. Even with a bald head, I didn't look "sick," but the combination of both really affected me.

- make an ugly sweater -

S.L. • Chemotherapy is the practice of poisoning the body at just low enough levels that it won't kill a person but hopefully kills everything else. I suggest finding a hobby that's possible to do while your blood is turning to toxic sludge in your veins, like listening to audiobooks or bad crocheting. Then at the end at least you'll have a terribly-made afghan.

- to wig or not to wig? -

T.H. • Speaking of hair loss, I bought an expensive natural hair wig that my insurance company paid for and I wore exactly once. I would not recommend a wig to most women because they are exceedingly uncomfortable. Instead, splurge on a soft knit cap. I bought one made of cashmere and it was like wearing a kitten on my head. It was wonderfully comfortable and kept my head warm at night through the coldest part of my treatment.

Hive Chemotherapy Tips:

• Drink your water, Pedialyte, Ensure, broth. Stay hydrated!

• Take your nausea meds.

• Sleep, sleep, and more sleep.

• Let people help.

Handle With Care

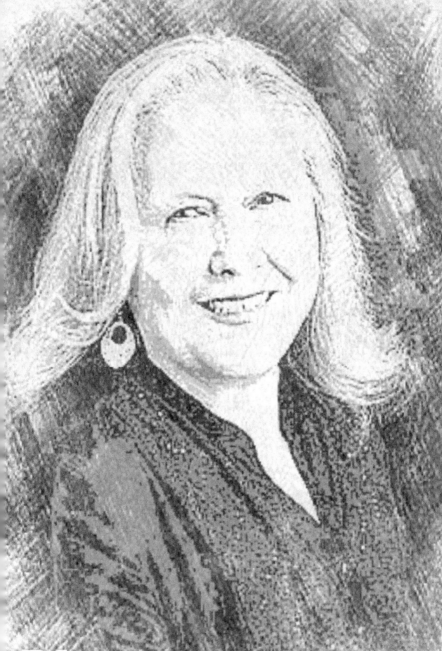

Diana

Radiation

If it's considered right in your particular case, then radiation therapy is where your radiation oncologist enters the scene, developing their treatment plan for you. Before the first radiation treatment, your breast will be mapped. This involves a CT scan so the radiation oncologist can map the treatment area to determine precisely where the beams of high-intensity radiation will be delivered. Radiation therapy is often given after a lumpectomy to ensure any remaining cancer cells will be killed.

Once the mapping is performed, a technician will tattoo small dots in the area to use as markers for precision. Six weeks; thirty-five treatment sessions, given at the same time each day; is standard.

Internal radiation therapy, or brachytherapy, is a more recent method of internal radiation therapy in which radiation seeds are placed in the body near the tumor. This is a newer technique that doesn't involve the daily treatments, and it is becoming more common.

The Hive weighs in on radiation:

- *about those radiation sunburns* -

Carrie • The worst part about radiation is that it's every day. Every Monday through Friday. Every freaking weekday. Treatment doesn't take long at all; in fact, your commute will probably suck up more of your time than getting zapped. It doesn't hurt; it's not scary; and, if you're lucky, they'll play music for you.

But it's every weekday. Without fail. Good skin care is key to getting through this as comfortably as possible.

Lavetta • Because of the burns, the most painful experience I had through everything that I've gone through was the radiation. I had to wear things like soft T-shirts, because I couldn't stand anything touching me. What I did, I cut some of the T-shirts up—because the white cotton T-shirts are very soft —and I would just put that under my arms and armpit and just wear it like that all day, my little cushion.

Ayanna • If I had to tell anyone anything, it would be that radiation hurts. But it does heal and your skin does lighten. As of today, it's still darker than the other side, but it's not so bad. If you have to work during treatment and you have a limited amount of time off, please save some hours for after your third or fourth radiation treatment just in case the pain is unbearable.

- *small comfort* -

Margaret • Biafine topical cream was an absolute godsend for my dark, ugly radiation sunburn. Once I began applying it to the area of the fold underneath my breast, the nasty burn began to heal within a few days. It felt like some kind of magic to me.

Diana • Once the skin starts to open—because mine did—I would go and get the surgical pads that they sell at Walgreen's or CVS—or wherever I could get them—and I would put Aquaphor or aloe vera cream on my body, and then I would put the pads on.

Handle With Care

And then the corsets that they give you after your mastectomy—which are tight—if it moves, then it was okay because the pad was there to catch the excess fluid.

Lavetta • My doctor did prescribe a cream for the burns. It didn't really help though. My skin just had to basically heal itself, because the skin was broken. It was like third-degree burns, it looked like to me. It was very painful under my armpits because the radiation hit me there, and in the area of my breast.

- *radiation implants* -

Christina • I only had radiation the first time I was diagnosed with what they called, back in 1997, "radiation implants." The implants went through a long needle going from one side of the breast to the other. Those radiation implants were placed for two weeks while at the hospital, and I couldn't have visitors for more then ten minutes at a time. I also had a shield in front of my hospital room door to shield anybody going into my room.

- *about radiation fatigue* -

T.H. • People will tell you that radiation causes fatigue. And it may, but for me, the fatigue with chemo was so awful, I never really noticed it with radiation. What I did notice was persistent mild nausea. My radiation oncologist assured me that wasn't due to radiation, but I've talked to enough cancer patients who claim the same thing, that I'm not sure my oncologist is right. I took my anti-nausea meds left over from chemo, and they helped.

S.L. • Radiation did not give me superpowers: One star. I would not radiate again.

- *like Mom said, take your nap!* -

Carrie • Listen to your body. I know that phrase is used over and over again, but truly, I napped more in the five weeks of radiation than I did in five years. I was exhausted, and my body just needed that rest. I didn't even have a choice but to listen to it. People just need to know that it's okay to rest. If you need to take that nap, take it. People like me—it was really difficult to be a bump on a log, but that's what I needed to do. So I say be prepared to nap, and don't feel bad about it!

Diana • Rest is important. Don't force yourself to do anything. Listen to your body. If your body is saying, "I'm miserable," then rest. That's the most important to me was getting rest, and eating when you can eat—if you feel like eating. Even though it's only like five minutes per time, the whole process, once you're in there and you're strapped in and stuff, it still saps you. It just totally saps you, and I was exhausted.

Margaret • After the sixty-mile roundtrip commute in traffic to my daily radiation treatments, I was ready for a nap when I returned home. An hour to an hour and a half (maybe two?) gave me the recharge I needed. (Plus, naps are almost better than tacos.)

- a little stretch here and there -

T.H. • Another thing I want to mention that isn't really related to radiation but impacted me at this time is lack of range of motion. If you need a mastectomy, your shoulder won't move the way it did before. You may have very limited range. You need to be able to get your arms over your head before you start radiation, so do some gentle stretching as soon as your surgeon okays it.

The other thing I would recommend investing in is a decent back scratcher, because your skin will itch in places you can no longer reach. You'll thank me for it.

- didn't have it (but wish I did) -

Kayte • I didn't get radiation. I wanted it, though. It may sound weird, but I wanted as much treatment as I could possibly get, so that I could prevent a recurrence that much more. My oncologist said the radiation wasn't needed, though, because of my bilateral mastectomy. So if you are offered radiation, don't be too disappointed. It just means that you're fighting that recurrence possibility that much harder! Yes, there are side effects, but I believe they are worth it in the long run.

- taking the short view -

Margaret • Treatment number one felt daunting—the first of thirty-five—but as with any really big challenge in life, it helped for me to take it one day at a time. Before I knew it—even though it seemed impossible in the beginning—the six weeks were up, and I was moving on to the next phase of treatment (and life). For me, I seized on the little things like small acts of kindness—the older man at the check-in desk with the big smile and contagious laugh —or my technicians who welcomed me each day—friendly, courteous, and attentive. I found myself actually missing them at the end of our time together.

Hive Radiation Tips:

• Aquaphor, Biofine, aloe vera gel, and Vitamin E oil for the burns.

• Naps. Often! (Did we mention to take lots of naps?)

• Soft clothing—cotton T-shirts or cloth diapers—in the radiation areas.

• Listen to your body.

• Breathe.

Handle With Care

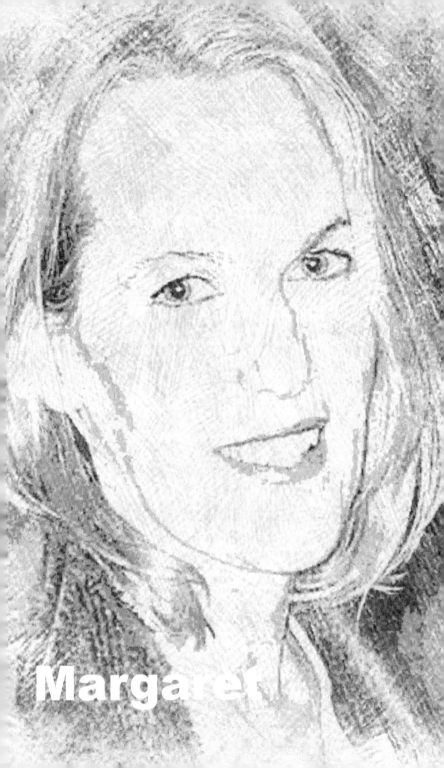
Margaret

Reconstruction

To reconstruct or not? Now, that is the Million-Dollar Question. If we choose to do so, do we opt to have tissue expanders placed during surgery to then be filled with saline injections over time, stretching the skin, and having the temporary expanders swapped later for the permanent implants?

Do we choose a more complicated flap procedure which involves taking skin from the back or abdomen and injecting fat tissue to rebuild, often yielding a more natural look and feel?

Do we opt not to reconstruct and use prosthetics?

Nothing at all?

Each has its pros and cons, and the Hive has many thoughts about this weighty (um, delicate?) topic, as well as what some of us think of our reconstructed chests and the complicated emotions that go along with them.

- *no rush* -

Carrie • Don't make any rash decisions. You don't have to have reconstruction, and most people aren't going to say that to you. Going flat is a real option. Staying with one breast is an option. And I think it's important to find a surgeon that you trust and feel comfortable with so that you can rely on what they think is best for your body type.

Not everybody is necessarily a candidate for every type of reconstruction, and I think people don't realize that. For example, a DIEP [Deep Inferior Epigastric Perforator artery] flap procedure isn't an option for everybody. So I think take your time, and get multiple opinions, if you can, from different surgeons. Then wait a while.

I know some people get immediate reconstruction, and if that is what they need, that's great. But for those who are on the fence, I say wait until you have a total peace about it, because there's no rush.

T.H. • Reconstruction was really important to me, but I have a number of friends in my support group who decided against it. They love their flat chests, sleeping on their stomachs, and not worrying about wearing a bra for the first time in their adult lives.

- it's not going to be the same -

T.H. • If reconstruction is something you feel strongly about, just temper your expectations. Your reconstructed boob will never look like the one you lost and will be a far cry from the one you still have, if you only had a single mastectomy. You have options, including implants or using your own skin and body fat to create a more realistic-looking breast. There is a longer recovery time for the non-implant route, but many women opt for one of these due to the look and feel.

Handle With Care

- *faux nipples or tattoos?* -

T.H. • Something else to factor in is nipples or no nipples. I chose a surgical option, and I hate it. It doesn't look anything like the one I have. There are amazing tattoo artists who can create very realistic-looking nipples. Or go all out and have your scars covered with vines, flowers, or something else that makes you feel beautiful. In most cases, the skin on your breast is numb, so at least it doesn't hurt!

- *more complete (for me)* -

Christina • My first cancer diagnosis, I did not opt to get reconstruction because I was very young and came from a very low-income family and had not been able to afford anything of that nature. (And, of course, I did not know that those procedures were covered under the insurance.) This made me feel very-self conscious about my body, and I had very low self-esteem. The second time, I opted for reconstruction. Being forty-five years old at the time of my second diagnosis, I did not care that much about my breast being gone, but it still made me feel incomplete. I felt like there was something missing from me that made me a complete women.

- *no reconstruction* -

Lavetta • When I was originally diagnosed in 2016, I had to wait a year after I finished radiation to even be considered for reconstruction. I had gone ahead and set it up and had my surgery date to have the surgery done. The day that I was going through my pre-op appointment, that was the day that I found out my cancer was back and I was diagnosed with Stage IV.

So I decided against it; I didn't want to go through any surgery. I use a prosthesis on the right side where they removed my breast.

I'm happy that I didn't go through the surgery, because there would have been more recovery time. And more surgery—because it takes more than one. You may have to go back for one or two more surgeries. So I decided against it, and I'm okay with that.

Diana • It wasn't important for me to have reconstruction. I talked to my surgeon and some of the other nurses, and they told me about the complications; that there can be complications. I said, "You know what? I've had complications enough with what I'm dealing with right now." And my surgeon said, "You can have it done later. It's going to be a little more painful because you don't have the expanders." And I said, "Well, that's okay. Boobs are not important to me. Life is important to me." End of story. Still, to this day, I don't regret it. I don't regret it at all.

Gina • I haven't had it. I had full intentions of doing it, but when I was first diagnosed, I was overwhelmed with having to make all of these decisions. You see your plastic surgeon, you see your surgeon, and it's like, "What do you want to do?" "What do you want to do?"

Handle With Care

I was so overwhelmed. I didn't want to be stressed out over it, so I told myself, I'm not going to force myself to make a decision at this moment, and it's my choice.

Ayanna • Still deciding if it's for me. So right now I'm flat.

- it's complicated -

Margaret • I have mixed feelings about my reconstruction. After my bilateral mastectomy, I opted to have tissue expanders placed, with a second surgery six months down the road to swap the expanders for permanent saline implants. Afterward, while I am grateful to have something on my chest that helps my clothes hang right and makes me a little less aware that something is missing, I sometimes wish I hadn't gone the reconstruction route. In the seven years since my surgery, I've often felt discomfort— especially at night. Sleep is often difficult or awkward because of positional limitations. So... It's complicated for me.

S.L. • I think I'm glad I did it, but I also think about reversing it every day. It's not a replacement. They're not mine. They're like... Something grafted on by an alien. They're not like the real thing, they're hard to fit into clothes—they don't squish correctly—and as an athlete I wonder if I would have lost as much of what's important to me if I hadn't had it done.

But on the plus side, I like that I think I look amazing in a black tie gown, and I might be just vain enough that I care. And I think that's okay, too. There's no shame or judgment in any of the choices here.

- *multiple surgeries* -

Kayte • I've had three, so far. I know that probably sounds a little excessive, but they were all worth it to me. The first one was to swap out the tissue expanders for implants. I thought I wanted to be bigger in size. Before being diagnosed, I was a small B cup and definitely a bit saggy after having breastfed both of my children for a total of eighteen months. So I wanted to be a full C cup, and "nice and perky." But the implants were very firm, and I felt too heavy, and one of them was off to the side too much. I'd feel it with my arm, when walking. So I knew I needed a redo.

The second time around, the implant that was bugging me was moved 2cm towards the center of my chest, and nipples were created out of my own skin. But they flattened out eventually, and you can hardly see them now.

- *third time's the charm (maybe?)* -

Kayte • The third time was a different plastic surgeon who gave me different, smaller, softer implants. But they are under the muscle, and any time I flex my pecs, they quickly turn into shriveled-up raisins. I also have a lot of scar tissue that is tight and painful when working out. So I might have yet another redo coming up. I'm still trying to decide on that. My best advice is to take it step by step and do what feels best for you and what will make you the happiest. Reconstruction is such a personal decision, and what is right for you could be completely wrong for one of your friends.

- *social stigma* -

Diana • When people found out that I wasn't going to have reconstruction and I wasn't going to have the implants put in, some women would actually say to me, "Well, what if you meet a man?"

I would say, "What if I meet a man? If I meet a man, then he would have to love me for me, with or without boobs. It's not the boob that he's going to love."

Carrie • My surgeon who gave me my results had the sweetest, kindest, most gentle spirit. He said, "Honey, you're forty. You're going to have reconstruction." Again, well intentioned, but he planted that in my brain, and I was in such a buzz with the news that I was like, "Okay, we'll just do the one for now."

Because I had asked, "Can we just take them both?" And he said, "You're going to have reconstruction, you should have the plastic surgeon do it." So I automatically went with that. But I think had I done the double mastectomy versus a single initially, I may not have gone on to have reconstruction. Because I had only a single mastectomy, and it was just awkward with a prosthesis, I felt obligated, if you will. Like, "Right now, I've got to do it," and I wish it would have been presented to me as an option not to.

Margaret • After talking to other women who've chosen not to go for reconstruction, I've learned that there is a kind of social stigma or pressure when a woman chooses not to reconstruct. Women who've opted not to often face pushback from family members and friends. Sometimes they feel guilt, or as if they're being judged about this very personal choice.

There should absolutely not be any judgment when a woman decides not to choose reconstruction. We each need to be able to make our own choice about what makes the most sense for us, for our lives, and our own happiness.

So what have we learned about Reconstruction?

• Reconstruction is not one-size-fits all.

• Ask your plastic surgeon to see pictures of different types of reconstruction results.

• Don't feel pressured to conform to society's view of what our bodies "should" look like.

• It's okay not to reconstruct.

• Take your time.

Handle With Care

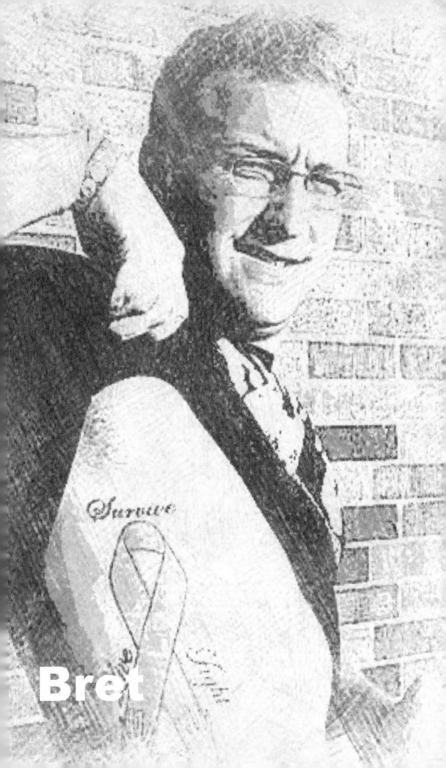

Survive

Bret

Men, Too

Male breast cancer is too often left out of the general discussion of breast cancer. Because of the lower rate of occurrence in the male population and scant public awareness, it's not uncommon for a man dealing with a breast cancer diagnosis to feel isolated, especially while sitting in a mammography room decorated with pink ribbons, designed and geared toward women.

Although the rate of occurrence in men is much less common, it doesn't feel rare—not when it's happening to you; not when it's happening to one of the men in your life.

Tragically, because of the lack of awareness on the subject, men often go undiagnosed until their cancer has progressed and has become more complicated to treat.

The good news is that there are groups out there for guys dealing with breast cancer offering moral support as well as being dedicated to raising awareness. If a man in your life receives a breast cancer diagnosis, he does not have to go it alone.

There is much more that needs to be done in this area, especially as far as public consciousness-raising and general knowledge, so we talked with Bret Miller, co-founder of MaleBreastCancerCoalition.org to find out a little bit about male breast cancer.

What do you want the world to know about male breast cancer?

Bret: That men have breasts too. Men need to know that although they don't have a physical breast like a woman's, they still have breast tissue and can be diagnosed with breast cancer.

Symptoms of male breast cancer can include:

• A painless lump or thickening in your breast tissue

• Changes to the skin covering your breast, such as dimpling, puckering, redness, or scaling

• Changes to the nipple, such as redness or scaling, or a nipple that begins to turn inward

• Discharge from the nipple

Types of male breast cancer:

• Cancer that begins in the milk ducts—ductal carcinoma, which is the most common form of male breast cancer.

• Cancer that begins in the milk-producing glands—lobular carcinoma. (This type is rare in men because they have few lobules in their breast tissue.)

• Other, rarer types of breast cancer that can occur in men include Paget's disease of the nipple, and inflammatory breast cancer.

Handle With Care

How old were you when you were diagnosed?

Bret: I was twenty-four years old.

[Fact: Male breast cancer is most common in older men, although it can occur at any age.]

How was your cancer discovered?

Bret: I was seventeen, watching TV, when I did a lean-back stretch and scratch across my chest and came across this lump directly below my right nipple.

[Fact: Men can receive a mammogram, or other imaging scan, just as a woman can.]

["Most cases of male breast cancer will present with an obvious breast mass, which is often behind the nipple. Sometimes, it will present as a mass in the upper outer portion of the breast or with nipple changes (ulceration, discharge, inversion)." (From Breast360.org)]

Does male breast cancer run in your family? Is there a genetic component?

Bret: There is no one else in my family with male breast cancer. There are twelve female cousins on my mom's side of the family with breast cancer.

[Fact: Some men inherit abnormal or mutated genes from their parents that increase the risk of breast cancer. Mutations in one of several genes, especially the BRCA2 gene, put you at greater risk of developing breast and prostate cancers.]

[Because of the low rate of occurrence in men, yearly mammograms are not recommended; however, physical examination by a doctor and regular breast self-examinations are.]

What treatment did you receive?

Bret: I first had the lump removed—a lumpectomy—on April 27, 2010. I received the call from the doctor the next day—not asking if I was sitting down or to come in; that there were things we needed to discuss. He just straight up over the phone told me that the preliminary pathology results say it's breast cancer, but that he would read the report and get back to me in three to five days.

I went with a second opinion and different doctor. That led to a mastectomy of my right breast and four rounds of chemotherapy. Between the lumpectomy and last day of chemotherapy, I missed eight days of work.

What words of wisdom would you share with a man diagnosed with breast cancer?

Bret: You are not alone. You may feel that at first, you might feel emasculated, but it will pass. There are many of us out here who will help. You can call on us with any questions.

Handle With Care

What resources are out there for men with breast cancer?

Bret: Visit **malebreastcancercoalition.org** to learn more about male breast cancer and read the stories of men who've gone through male breast cancer.

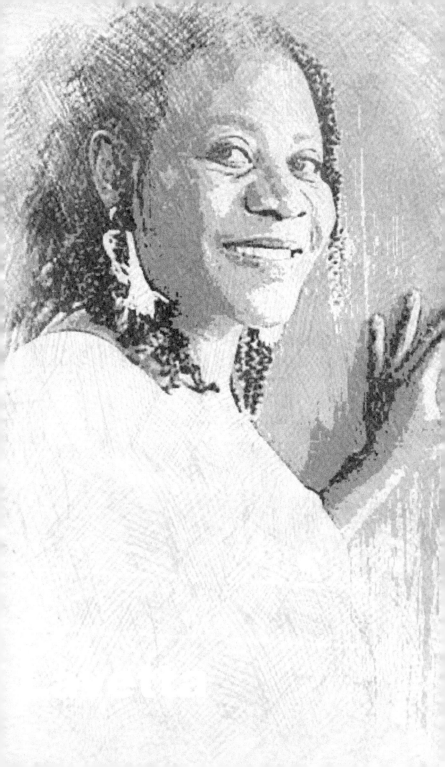

Self-Care

If a diagnosis of breast cancer teaches us anything, it is that we need to take some time for a little self-care. What that looks like may be different for each of us and can be anything from a soothing massage to a few moments of quiet during a hectic day. After everything our bodies have gone through—surgery; medications; chemotherapy; radiation; stress, stress, and more stress—we need to give ourselves a break. Every day, if possible, whether five minutes or thirty. (Or even an hour. Live large!)

Here are a few ways the Hive takes care of themselves:

- *I am my priority* -

T.H. • This was probably the toughest one for me. As women, we're used to taking care of everyone else and letting our own care fall to the wayside. In fact, that may be why I didn't notice my symptoms sooner. But making yourself a priority is key in this battle. Not only should you accept help when it's offered, don't be afraid to ask for what you need. You can't do everything. Not only won't you have the energy, but depending on the drugs you're given, you may not even be legally allowed to drive. Going out in public can put your health at extreme risk when your white blood cell count is at its lowest.

Carrie • Take a nap!

- *treat yourself* -

Carrie • I think that for me personally, I grew up with a mom who's always worked full time and a dad who's always worked really hard, and that's just the culture of our society. Work, work, work. Nobody tells you or teaches you that it's important to stop and take a deep breath. It's important to work out and really keep your body as strong as possible. It's not even about being skinny, it's about being healthy.

People really need to just value their body the same way you take care of your car, you know, with your regular oil changes and your tune-ups. We need to take care of ourselves, and people don't think about it until they get sick. It's so good for prevention, for maintenance, for recovery, and for hopefully helping to prevent a recurrence.

- *sparkly nail polish* -

Kayte • Besides going through the obvious steps of listening to your doctors and their treatment plans they have for you, eating very healthy, and getting plenty of sleep, I think it is also important to find something that makes you feel pretty or lifts your spirits a little. My thing that made me happy was getting my nails done. My sister-in-law would come over to my house, sometimes weekly, with her gel kit and come up with lots of fun colors and designs for them. It always made me feel just a little bit better, even on my bad days. Sure, I was bald, flat-chested, and feeling like crap, but my hands were fun to look at!

Handle With Care

- *playing in the dirt* -

Diana • I had this big tree in the back yard, and because I love potting—working with dirt and planting plants—my friend put a table and chairs under the tree for me. (This was during the time I was going through chemo.) People had given me a bunch of plants during that time, and I needed to take the plants out of the cutesy pots and put them in bigger pots. I had a selection of potting soil, and that's the only thing that would calm me. Just soothe me. So I would put my gloves on, and my friend would have me in hats, and I would be covered in long-sleeved shirts, and we would sit out there under the tree, so I wasn't in direct sun.

During this time, I knew I couldn't just work in the dirt because of possible germs, so I always used gloves. Before I would even put the gardening gloves on, I would put plastic gloves on first, just to be doubly safe. It was fantastic. You're one with the earth. It's soothing and calming. You're now releasing whatever is going on inside you—you're releasing it because you're thinking about something else.

- *be kind to yourself* -

T.H. • Let your body rest, pamper yourself, and take advantage of your good days. You'll normally feel great on the day of chemo and then again about ten days after, though you'll start to feel a little better every day after about four days post-chemo. While you may start to feel like yourself again, don't overdo it. Use those days to treat yourself to a lunch out with a friend, get a massage, if you are comfortable with that, or try an alternative treatment to deal with your side effects. Many women swear by acupuncture.

Take a yoga class—there are a number of these specifically for women undergoing breast cancer treatment. Or give meditation a try. Or try your hand at painting. Just focus on yourself during this time, because once you're done with treatment, life will quickly return to the crazy pace it was before.

Ayanna • Take care of yourself, even if it means someone will be upset with you. Say "No" if it means your peace of mind will be sacrificed.

- avoid comparisons -

Margaret • It's easy to fall into the trap of comparing ourselves to others and questioning why we haven't bounced back from surgery as fast as our friend did, or being frustrated by not having energy to work during treatment. For me, my recovery after my mastectomy went a lot more slowly than other women I talked to. (I was definitely not one of those people able to drive ten days out from surgery.) My body needed more time.

We sometimes need to remind ourselves to be patient; the healing process is a little different for each of us.

Be kind to yourself.

- release the negative influences -

Lavetta • I shun negative people, even if they're my family members. I do, because I can't have that in my life.

Handle With Care

Margaret • As I was going through my treatment, I learned to avoid overly negative people like the plague. Connect with people who fill your spiritual fuel tank, who make you laugh. If you find yourself the victim of a one-sided conversation—the other person is monopolizing things and not letting you participate—find any excuse to extricate yourself. (Also filed under the category: Life is too short.)

- sometimes self-care is no self-care -

S.L. • Self-care... I didn't try for any, at least not specifically. It would have been an additional stress. I was just focused on getting through. What I did try for was doing some work when I could, which made me feel more like myself. It wasn't much, but all I wanted was to feel normal.

- mind and body care -

Christina • I am focusing now on pleasing myself more and enjoying life to the fullest. I try to travel when I can and not sweat the little things anymore. I have found my inner peace through prayer.

Lavetta • During treatment, the only self-care that I did was spiritual self-care. I prayed, and I read my Bible. I was still going to church, so that filled my soul.

After I recovered, that's when I started going to the gym more. Also, I changed my eating habits. I do yoga, meditation, and I went from a vegetarian to a vegan diet, and that's what I'm doing now.

My main self-care is meditation. Every day. And making sure that I'm getting the proper rest that I need.

Kay • My self-care: Days without obligations. Being present in the moment. Disconnecting with travel.

Gina • Other than watching what I eat, and trying to keep moving, for me part of self-care has to do with not just the physical part but the mental part also. I had to start going to therapy—doing those types of things that I had never done my whole life. Now that I do them, it does help me to kind of ground myself, and I'm more able to process things a little bit better than I was after it all. To me, I think everybody needs to go see a therapist at one point or another.

A good part of the self-care is just part of that: Live, laugh, and do things that make your heart happy.

So what have we learned about Self-Care?

• Give yourself a break.

• Try not to sweat the small stuff.

Handle With Care

• Don't underestimate the power of a good mani/pedi or massage.

• Find something that helps re-charge and replenish your soul. We all need a boost, especially during treatment.

• Don't forget to laugh. Find something dumb/silly/juvenile to watch, and laugh out loud.

• Turn the music up.

• Be kind to yourself.

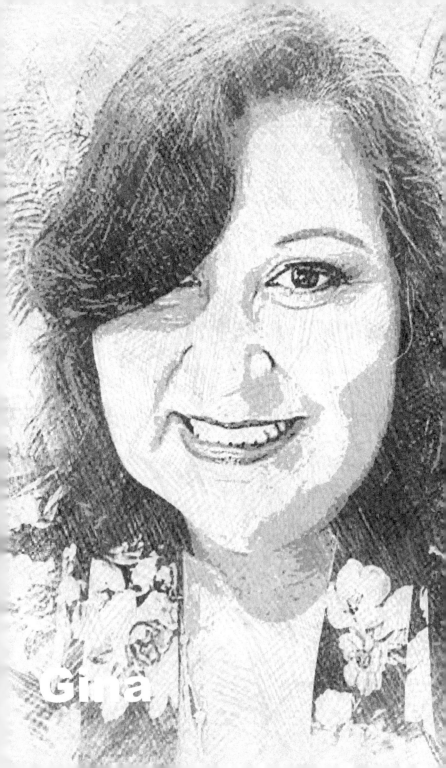

Words of Hope / What Gave Us Hope

"We must accept finite disappointment, but never lose infinite hope." ~ *The Rev. Dr. Martin Luther King, Jr.*

Sometimes it was a word or two of comfort—a smile in an unexpected place; the kindness of a stranger; a hand on the shoulder giving us that little push we needed to keep going. The promise of a new day.

Maybe it was our own internal pep talks:

"I'm going to get through this. Today, at least."

"Okay, maybe for the next half hour."

"Maybe for the next five minutes."

"This minute. I will definitely get through this one minute..."

One day, one step, one increment of time.

The Hive weighs in on the topic of things that motivated us to keep going:

- *my kids* -

Carrie • My hope was living long enough to see my kids off on their own. As a single mom, knowing I was all they had, I just had to hold on to the hope that they were still needing me enough, that the universe was going to let me live. I had that peace that I was going to live, and my motivation was all my kids, biological and the others.

- *those who walked the path before us* -

Kay • Hearing that other MBCs [metastatic breast cancer] have outlived their prognosis has helped me to see endless possibilities. Also, learning that the mind has a will that can carry our bodies out of precarious situations.

Margaret • Something I latched onto when I was very much a terrified mess was hearing from a long-term breast cancer survivor who called me out of the blue, something she did often for others as a volunteer with the American Cancer Society. Hearing her story about long-term survival was the exact thing I needed to hear. Her words gave me hope, helping to ease my many fears. I soon learned, the more people I spoke to: Cancer survivors and thrivers are everywhere around us.

Kayte • I think the thing that has helped me the most, after being diagnosed, was getting to hear about all the survivors who have been cancer-free for decades upon decades now, after their initial diagnosis. They are happy and living their lives in a fierce, passionate, honest way. Every time I meet a new one—or even hear of someone, like a friend of a friend—who is doing well thirty years later, my heart is so happy.

Christina • My children gave me hope, as well as my grandson, but mostly all the women I saw going through it who beat it.

T.H. • With inflammatory breast cancer, I wasn't finding much in the way of hope online. Not at first anyway. All I found were the terrifying statistics. But when I discovered an online IBC support group, I digitally met dozens of long-term survivors who have been living with no evidence of disease (NED) for years or decades. These long-term survivors were treated before current advancements, giving me even more hope.

A local support group cropped up from that worldwide group. Meeting women in person has been a blessing. We laugh together, cry together, and support each other. Hearing about their battles and how they've lived their lives to the fullest since their diagnosis gave me the courage to do the same. I'm not living my life as if I'll live forever, because no one does, but I'm also not going through the motions like "dead woman walking." I take advantage of every opportunity presented to me, including a once-in-a-lifetime chance to visit Italy with friends a year after my treatment was completed. But I'm also planning long-term, because there's a chance I WILL be here to see those plans come to fruition.

- *medical advances* -

Kayte • I love reading about new treatments, and in particular, the new medications that are showing real promise for our future. As a nurse case manager, I research many of these medications during my typical work day, and I am always excited when coming across a new one that shows promise.

- *positivity* -

Diana • Positivity, just thinking that "this too shall pass" is what got me through. I never, in my wildest dreams, thought I would ever survive this. There were times that I felt so awful that I was thinking "I have to make it. I just have to absolutely make it, but I can't even raise my head."

Ayanna • It will get better!

- *and prayer* -

Diana • Prayer. I'm a great believer in prayer, and the day of my surgery, I had no fear. I could feel everyone's prayers. When they had me in pre-op and were getting me ready for surgery... I can't explain it. There was just a peacefulness all around me I could feel like a shield. And my girlfriends—you could tell they were very nervous. You could see their faces, and I was comforting them. And it was like, "No, don't worry. I'm just fine." I kept telling them, "I'm going to be fine."

I had no fear, and I know that was because of prayer. Prayer and positivity. Thinking "This too, I'm going to pass it. I'm going to come out the other side. I don't care how I'm going to get there, but I'm going to get there."

- *hope? nope* -

S.L. • I didn't use hope. I used anger. Healthy? Maybe not, but it was what I had. Cancer treatment is dehumanizing. It removes agency; it warps life and relationships. I didn't have a say in how bad it was, but I didn't want to let it win in taking over my life. I lost that battle... Is this hopeful? This doesn't feel hopeful. I guess I'm still angry.

- *my faith* -

Gina • I think my faith, out of everything, is what gave me the most hope. I just think that the minute I was diagnosed, I felt that instead of being angry, instead of seeking blame or asking the Lord "Why?" or feeling that sense of guilt that I wasn't taking care of myself, I think I just kind of stepped back and said, "Okay, Lord."

So for me, I think at that moment I'm like, "All right, I have cancer. So what's my story going to be? What am I going to show others through it?"

– & –

So what have we learned about Hope?

• Use what works for you, whether it's talking to long-term survivors and thrivers; prayer; meditation; your children; your faith.

• It's helpful to be able to train our focus on something beyond ourselves and our bodies to take us out of our own pain and worry; redirect, regroup, and walk on—to the next challenge.

• In the bleakest of times, we still have the stars in the sky and the sun on our faces.

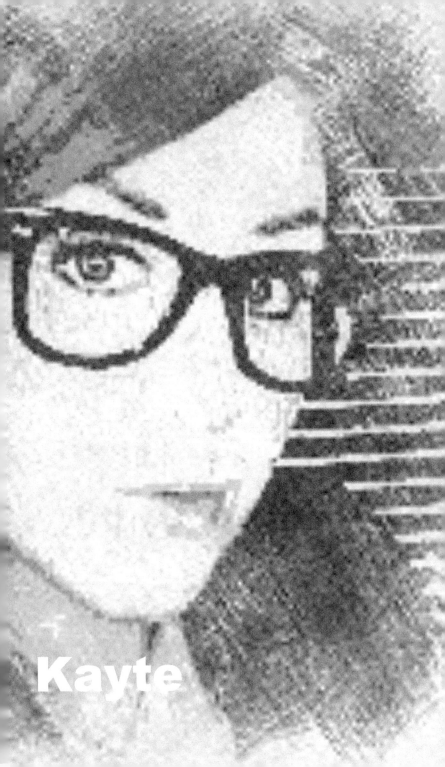
Kayte

Finding Our Power / Inspiration

"At the end of the day, we can endure much more than we think we can." ~ Frida Kahlo

Dealing with the complicated emotions and physical challenges that accompany a cancer diagnosis can leave us feeling anything but powerful as we struggle with what our new normal looks like; wondering how we'll resume our work, if we've been off on leave; worrying about how people will see us and treat us; what our love lives will be like with our scars and forever-changed bodies. Just getting through treatment itself is a major accomplishment.

Power, inspiration, and strength come in many forms. For some of us, seeing others overcome more challenging physical obstacles helped us find our own strength. For others, it was our children and having to function for them, because we had no other option but to get up and get them ready for school. This also applies to furry children, who shove wet noses in our laps when we're trying to rest, letting us know the dog dish is in need of re-filling. There is no ignoring their pleas, especially when they're capable of standing there for several hours, sending focused laser beams at you as you're trying to sleep. So you get up, you feed your dog, and then you feel like maybe brushing your teeth and washing your face. Dogs are tricky like that. So are people.

The Hive talks about the things that gave us that extra little nudge we needed:

- *helping others find a silver lining* -

Carrie • As I started treatment, I met so many people—both in the treatment center and online—and I started hearing how much worse they had it. Whether it was their diagnosis, their complications, lack of family or friends. That's how I started kind of trying to help people see things from a different perspective and find that silver lining in their day, in their week, or in their diagnosis. It was kind of in that moment that I realized I was organically mentoring others while still in treatment, and that's when the whole CARE Project thing came up for me. That's when I knew I could help people.

- *our strengths* -

T.H. • I found inspiration and power in close friends and family. I created a private Facebook group to keep these people updated on my progress. I often didn't have the energy for phone calls, but people wanted to know how I was doing. This was a safe place for me to open up about what was happening. For obvious reasons, I didn't include my mother in this group, but continued to update her and my father in person or via direct text messages, excluding some of the brutal honesty that might have scared them. Within this online group I could bare it all.

Handle With Care

Ayanna • You will not know your strength until you have to use it, but... Believe me, you have it.

Kay • Finding my inner beast (or beast within). Realizing that the grit and tenacity I have is a gift in my survival.

- whatever works for you, do that -

S.L. • What got me through was my determination to return to my "normal" life afterward. I ended up not being able to do that—but I suppose I'm glad I had it as a motivator at the time. I also never lost my sense of humor, even though it got cynical, and I think that's important. Joking about cancer helps reclaim power from it. Use whatever you need to. Hang onto anything that helps. If it changes later, let it. If it doesn't, keep going with it. This is survival; do what works.

- the funny side -

T.H. • When I tried medical marijuana for the first time, I took too much and some of the posts I typed up in my private group while higher than a kite still make me laugh out loud.

My friends posted funny memes or jokes about breast cancer to keep me laughing. A sense of humor got me through some of the toughest times. I haven't posted an update in there in well over a year, but if things take a negative turn, it's a relief just knowing I have that safe space to break any bad news first and get the support I'll need.

- *people who touched our lives* -

Christina • I found my inspiration for becoming a mentor from my sweet angel Shannon Kristine Brown. She was my mentor, and she showed me what true love and strength really were. I want to believe that I have developed the power of caring and helping other survivors, which is what Shannon instilled in my heart and soul.

Lavetta • What inspired me most during the treatment was meeting other women that were going through the same thing that I was going through, in a different way. These women motivated me, they encouraged me, they inspired me to just keep doing what I was doing, to just keep going through treatment; that it was going to be over with soon. That's what inspired me most, my breast cancer support group that I attended during that time.

- *bald is beautiful* -

Carrie • In the very beginning of chemo, shaving my own head—or having my daughter do it—that was the most powerful I felt. Because you're so helpless, you're so out of control, that was something that made me think that I was powerful and a bit of a badass to walk around bald. I was like, "Yeah? What? I'm bald."

- *paying it forward* -

Kayte • After living through breast cancer and managing to put the puzzle pieces all back together, sometimes with the help of others, I am now inspired to help others with their pieces. And I have some amazing examples of women, who have journeyed before me, and then helped me along the way. Like Carrie, who started her own nonprofit to help fighters in need. And Margaret, whose written word has soothed so many souls. The people in my life who have wrapped their arms around me, in support and love, inspire me to do the same for as many as I possibly can. Still coming up with more ways I can do so. Participating in this book is one of them, though. I hope our words help you and make your day shine just a little bit brighter.

- *reading others' stories* -

Diana • My friends had brought me these books about being positive and inspirational—not about breast cancer, but stories where there were circumstances that people came out of—to see that there was hope.

- *telling our own stories* -

Gina • I think for me, I didn't really think I had any power. I actually felt powerless for a very long time. When it came to being able to outwardly show people that there is hope, being open with my struggles, being open with my fight, being open with my faith

—I think within all that, something happened to me, and I just realized because of all of it that people were paying attention and that I need to be very cognizant of the things that I was doing from that moment forward.

People have asked me to speak; people have asked me to mentor their loved ones; people have asked me to share my story. People have asked me to just do crazy stuff, and I feel like it's the craziest thing, but I'm going to do it, and I'm just letting it happen.

Margaret • When I was going through my recurrence, feeling awkward about openly discussing my bilateral mastectomy—and not enjoying the looks of pity I would get from well-meaning people—I started writing about the process and sharing my reflections on my blog. I wrote about the weirdness of my reconstruction (my "Frankenboobs"); the absurd things that made me laugh; the things that made me feel vulnerable; the things that were most important to me. The more I shared, the less self-conscious I became. So there was definitely a power, for me, in sharing.

So what have we learned about power and inspiration?

• We pay it forward by helping others going through what we've already been through.

• We can be our own hero by pushing ourselves out of our comfort zones to share and comfort others.

• Finding the humor in our own situations. By not taking ourselves too seriously, we're more likely to see the absurd. Laughter and tears are not that different, one often leads to the other.

• We are humans, social beings, and we find power in our connections with each other.

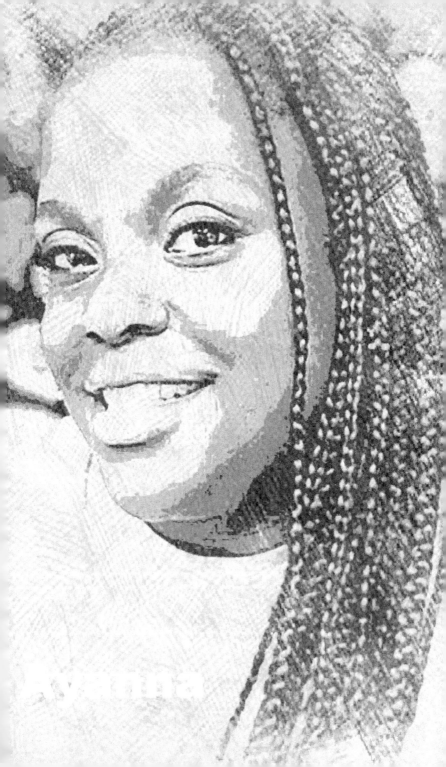

What Surprised Us

For so many of us—especially those of us with no family history of breast cancer and little experience with cancer in general—we didn't have a roadmap we could look to that laid out our immediate future. But since life has a tendency of throwing us curveballs—a cancer diagnosis being one big, fat, uninvited curveball—we learn along the way.

A few things about cancer surprised us, including who in our lives reached out (and who didn't), and just how much support we received from the most unexpected places.

From the kindness of strangers to the disappointment of long-term connections, the Hive talks about the things that surprised us:

- *you think you know people* -

Carrie • I think what surprised me the most was the amount of people—friends—that fell off, that left my life. You see all these commercials with all of these people and these heart-warming stories of "Oh, look at all these friends who shaved their heads in support."

You think all those people are going to be there—and it's great for all those people that have that—but I was stunned by the amount of people who withered away and have never come back, and the amount of other survivors I know that have experienced this same exact thing. I don't know what that is.

I think it's scary for friends to see us diagnosed as it brings about the realization they too could be diagnosed.

Lavetta • What surprised me the most was the friends who I thought were really my friends, some of them didn't come around, they didn't call, they didn't send a card. They didn't touch base with me at all. And some of the people, I thought we were really good friends! They just dropped off, and so I didn't bother to reach out to them anymore. That's what really surprised me the most, and it was kind of hurtful, too. These people, some of them had been in my life for years that I just didn't hear from them at all. That's what really surprised me.

- accepting help from others -

T.H. • What surprised me, and continues to even three years later, is the generosity of complete strangers. The community came out in force to support us. The effort was led by a couple of good friends of mine, but I was blown away by how many people I either had never met, or barely saw in passing, signed up to bring us food, offered to take me to appointments, or take the kids to and from school. Accepting help was hard. I've always been independent, waiting until my thirties to marry, doing most everything on my own after that since my husband travels so much. But even as stubbornly independent as I am, I had to admit I couldn't do it all on my own.

Handle With Care

- *perspective* -

Kay • Things that surprised me:

How much people cared about me and saw me as an inspiration.

The stigma around breast cancer.

The empathy I developed for women who don't have the resources to focus on cancer—financial means, social and familial support, access to health care and alternative medicine.

- *harsh financial reality* -

S.L. • My insurance was very good. The California unemployment system was not. They wouldn't let me file until I was firmly "disabled," at which point I was too sick to file. Then they took endless amounts of phone-chewing to get the claim processed and accused me of trying to scam the system. I am incredibly lucky to have close family members who fought all this for me. My family also applied for a number of grants that helped me stay out of debt while I couldn't work. I got a surprising and heartwarming amount of financial help, but there's absolutely no way I could have dealt with the logistics of any of it on my own.

The things they don't tell you about having cancer...

- *scanxiety is real* -

Margaret • Scanxiety (scan anxiety)—the fear or apprehension experienced by cancer patients over their next diagnostic scan and results—is a real thing. Also, even for longer-term survivors and thrivers, the heightened awareness we have of any new lumps, bumps, or pains, and the accompanying worry when we discover this new, fun thing on our body. (So many of us feel like we're turning into hypochondriacs because of this heightened awareness.)

About a year out from my first diagnosis, I ran to my oncologist's office after feeling a hard knot near my lumpectomy scar, afraid it was a new tumor. She did a quick exam, assuring me it was scar tissue. Sensing my worry, she eased my mind, telling me: "Come see me any time. You don't need an appointment." That helped, knowing she was there, available to me.

- *there is so much to learn* -

Christina • I was surprised at how many types or sub-types of breast cancer there are. I wish I had known what questions to ask the first time I was diagnosed as I know now.

- *learning the hard way* -

Ayanna • Doctors don't always know best.

Bret • What surprised me about my cancer experience was that very few men were talking about being diagnosed. It also was surprising to find that fewer "breast cancer foundations" were willing to help men.

- *if someone offers you help, take it* -

T.H. • Now that I'm on the other side of this and have had the chance to help others, I realize it wasn't a burden for them. People genuinely want to support one another. Sometimes it's hard to remember this when we hear name calling and childish behavior by our elected leaders. But the overwhelming majority of people have big hearts and want to help. If someone offers you help, take it. Even if doing so feels harder than fighting the disease itself.

- *a newer you* -

Kayte • When first diagnosed, it's very difficult to imagine your life after cancer. Like: How can you get back to the life you had prior to your diagnosis? But I have learned over time that you don't ever get back to that same "normal life" you once lived, even though you think you want to, at first. Because throughout your journey, you gain so much more empathy, wisdom, and respect for each and every day you are given, so returning to your old life is not only impossible, but, surprisingly, something you don't even want anymore.

You've upped your game to a superstar survivor who is ready to take on life in a whole new way.

- *our circle* - .

Gina • I think the biggest thing out of the surprises is you really do define your circle. It's pretty tight. You know who's who, you know who is genuine, and you have your circle. And, of course, you open it up to new people, and that was a surprise to me.

- *outlook* -

Margaret • All these years later, I am still genuinely surprised by how much breast cancer has changed my overall outlook on life. For the better. For instance, I tend to not take my health for granted or the health of the people close to me. And I know it's a cliche, but I honestly try to take time to enjoy the sunsets. (And my two cups of coffee a day, that too.) The little incredible everyday life things—I try to notice them and appreciate them.

Handle With Care

– & –

So what have we learned about what surprised us?

• While many of us had experiences with people drifting out of our lives—and this seems to be a universal phenomenon experienced by people dealing with a cancer diagnosis—we also made new friends and solidified existing relationships.

• Some people in our social networks stepped up in ways we least suspected.

• Help appeared, sometimes in the most unexpected forms.

• And we were more resilient than we realized.

• We surprised ourselves with just how incredible we are.

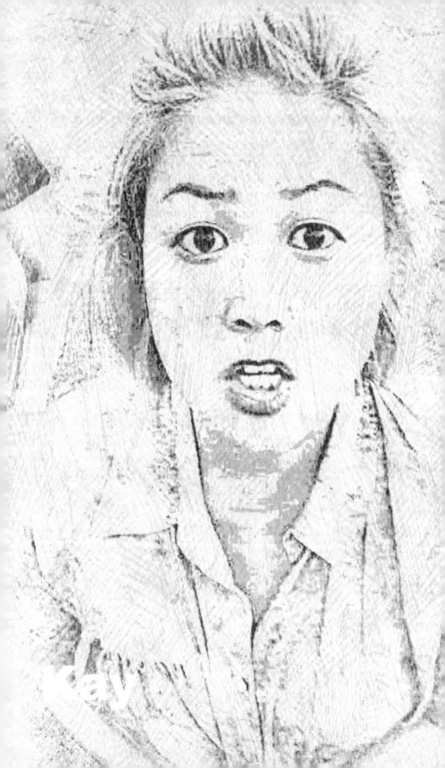

What We Don't Want to Hear

A truth universally acknowledged among those of us who've found ourselves dealing with a cancer diagnosis is, as sure as the Real Housewives franchise will continue to endure, folks will come out of the woodwork ready to give their unsolicited opinions about the miracle fruit we need to consume by the pound that will most definitely cure us; horror stories of terrible things that happened to their neighbor or great aunt with cancer; or simply ridiculous things that could have been left in the vault. Forever. And we will most likely want to smack them upside the head when they express these pearls of wisdom to us, but we won't. Because we're kind people. (Right? Sure we are.)

Here are a few things we sincerely do not want to hear:

- *free tummy tuck!* -

Carrie • "At least you got a tummy tuck." Because I had a DIEP flap reconstruction, everybody says that to me. "At least you got a tummy tuck out of it!"

Really? That's not what it feels like. Not what it feels like. I think I hate that.

- *don't say this* -

Kay • "You're not going to die."

- *or this* -

Lavetta • It was irritating, when they would say something like, "Oh, I have a cousin or a sister" or whoever, a relative or friend, "they had cancer, and they did this and they did that, and they're okay now." Or even they'd say, "They died."

T.H. • This is a broad category, because there are so many things we don't want to hear. We don't want to hear how your mom, sister, aunt, or cousin died of breast cancer, even though that is a big emotional part of your life. Being reminded that breast cancer is very much still a fatal disease for far too many doesn't help at this stage.

[Can we all agree on something? If you're reading this book, hold up your hand and say it with us: I will not talk about a loved one—aunt, uncle, cousin, great-grandmother, kindergarten teacher—who died of cancer with someone who is currently dealing with their own diagnosis. Not. Helpful.]

Handle With Care

- *unsolicited opinions* -

Kayte • Right after being diagnosed and sharing it on Facebook, I was surprised by how many people tried to give me advice—that I hadn't even asked for. So many people assumed because I was only thirty-three years old and diagnosed with cancer that I must have been living an unhealthy life prior to my diagnosis. It was like they needed to blame my cancer on something I had done wrong, I think? Because the mere thought of a very healthy young person getting cancer was probably pretty scary to hear about.

- *advice not needed!* -

Kayte • I was told that I shouldn't eat fast food anymore. And that I shouldn't drink soda anymore. And that I should start to exercise regularly. They didn't bother to ask me if I actually did those things. I wasn't into fast food at the time, and I definitely wasn't a soda drinker. I was into Cardio Barre and lots of water. I was very lean and muscly. I ate lots of vegetables and never touched red meat (which was yet another food they told me to stop eating). Kind of frustrating. But I decided to let it go and just realized that it was their fear that was making them give me this unneeded advice. Anyone can get cancer, even the people living healthy lifestyles.

- *call me!* -

Lavetta • I personally hated when someone told me "Call me!"

or "Let me know if you need anything." I couldn't stand that, and I can't even stand it now, you know? "If you need anything, just call me." Okay, if I call you and I tell you what I need, are you really going to deliver? That's a pet peeve of mine, but that's what it was for me.

Christina • "You are strong and will get through it." I also did not want to hear that God only sends this to the toughest.

- *free boobs! get them here!* -

Christina • One thing that was told to me the first time I was diagnosed, from my ex, is that God had sent me the cancer because I did something wrong.

I was also told, "Wow. Well, at least you'll be getting a free boob job."

T.H. • We don't want to hear "At least it was caught early," or "Hey, you get new boobs out of this."

Margaret • When someone would say, "At least you get a free boob job!" I had to stifle my punching impulses. (And I'm not a violent person. Really!) A mastectomy and reconstructive surgery does not equate to a free boob job. Not the same. Not the same. Not the same. So don't say it, people! Just don't.

Kayte • Another thing I didn't want to hear, which is probably the most common, was, "Well, at least you get a free boob job out of

Handle With Care

it!" Definitely didn't end up with a "boob job." More like a "You-can't-tell-that-anything-happened-to-me-if-I'm-wearing-a-sports-bra" job? Certainly not the same thing. Lots of scars, and no nipples to prove it. LOL.

- *blanket generalizations* -

Gina • I don't like when others simplify it. I had a lot of good friends say things that were very surprising to me:

"You got the good cancer."

"It's not as bad because you got breast cancer."

"Oh, now that chemo's over, you can get on with your life."

I don't like when people simplify it. I didn't think there was anything simple, by far, about anything that I went through. For me it was huge. It was very much a life-changer for me.

Bret • As a male, I don't want to hear statistics. I don't want to hear it is only one percent of breast cancer cases, and that there isn't enough research out there for men, so we are going to use this treatment that worked for women diagnosed with the same cancer and hope it works.

- *what? no reconstruction? gasp!* -

Diana • "How could you not go in and have reconstruction? How could you not take advantage of getting a nice pair of boobs?" (Not my close friends, but acquaintances.)

- *leave the conspiracy theories at home* -

T.H. • What I find infuriating is the number of people who told me, and continue to tell me, that cancer researchers aren't looking for a cure because they make too much money off of chemo. Yes, chemo is ridiculously expensive. Each of my six rounds was over $30,000. But to say that "Big Pharma" doesn't care and is hiding a cure is insulting to every researcher who has lost a loved one to this heinous disease. It says they care more about money than their own child, wife, mother.

It's so easy to look for a bad guy to blame, but the truth is, cancerous cells are in all of us. Every day our body finds, attacks, and kills cancer cells, until at some point, in some of us, it can no longer do the job. Yes, companies can be selfish and sometimes care about the bottom line more than people—just look at the recent opioid epidemic— but to claim that the entire pharmaceutical industry is behind a massive conspiracy doesn't help anyone fighting for their lives. In some ways it can even be harmful, especially when these same people will tell you there are natural cures that are being hidden from us. Because there are not. Not yet anyway. And if they are discovered, no one is going to hide them from us.

- *but your hair!* -

Diana • "Oh, don't you just hate that you lost your hair?"

It's like, "Why would you say that?"

- sometimes we're not strong, that's okay -

Carrie • I hated hearing all the "Just stay strong!" "Just stay positive!"

I wish I had had some coaching before. I wish I had a group like ours that would say to someone, "Hey, if someone says that to you, just know they're well intentioned. If it's really getting to you, stop them. Say, "I appreciate the sentiment, but it's not helpful right at the moment."

It's okay not to be strong all the time, it's okay not to be positive all the time. That's normal.

S.L. • "You're so strong."

"You're an inspiration."

"You're so brave."

"I could never do that."

Yes, you could, if you were forced to. None of us chose this. I didn't wake up one morning and think, "Oh, nice day for cancer. I think I'll become a role model." The best response I got when I told people my diagnosis was my friend who just said, "Balls." The best response I got when I revealed my health history to someone later was a friend who extended a fist bump and said, "Way to not die!" That works for me, but like anything else, it's individual. People who know you will hopefully know their audience and be able to say something that doesn't make you wish you were back under anesthesia so you didn't have to talk to them. Other people will mean well but be more exhausting than the treatment.

– *&* –

People don't set out to hurt us; they mean well. A big takeaway, though, from the collected wisdom of the Hive is that many comments are better left unsaid. That being said, we do have a few suggestions for family members, friends, and loved ones.

– *so what do we want to hear?* –

Carrie • "Let me know when your next appointment is. I'd love to drive you and tag along."

"I drove by your house and noticed your lawn needs to be cut. I'll stop by Saturday and do that."

"I know you're going to radiation daily for the next six weeks, so some of us got together and got you gift cards for gas! Here's one for each week."

"I'm taking my kids to the movies, and I'd like to pick yours up and take them with us. Can they be ready in an hour?"

"I'm ordering pizza for the family and want to order some for yours. What would they like? I'll have it delivered."

"What's a good day to swing by? I'd love to just sit and watch crap TV with you."

"I remember how much water I went through during chemo, trying to stay hydrated, so I left a case on your porch. Have your family bring it in for you."

"During chemo, my dentist told me to use Biotene mouthwash to prevent dry mouth and sores. I was at the drug store and picked some up for you. When can I deliver?"

Margaret • "I'm so sorry you're going through this. Do you feel like talking?"

Keep it simple. Be there. Don't disappear.

Also, if you send your friend with cancer a card, consider tucking a GrubHub gift certificate inside so they can order in when they're not feeling well enough to fix dinner.

When in doubt, send chocolate. (**Good** chocolate. None of that waxy stuff.)

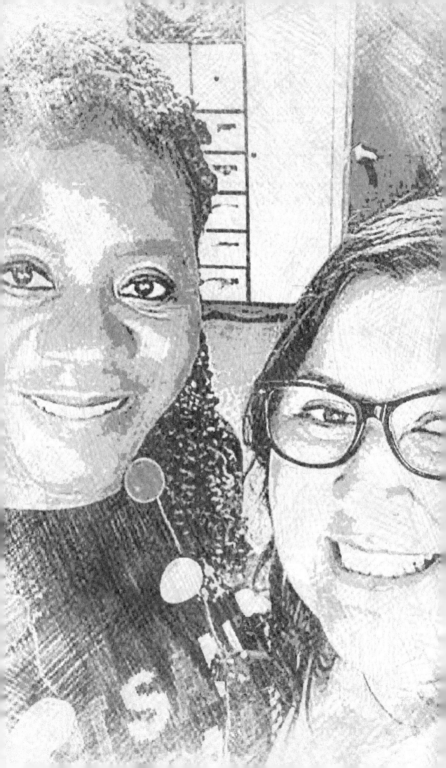

Support Groups

Support groups: Most communities have them, and if there isn't a formal breast cancer support group in your area, you'll probably be able to find at least a general cancer support community. And an up side to living in the Social Media Age—we have a multitude of ways to connect with others going through similar situations, whether it's with Facebook groups, Twitter chats, Google Hangouts, subReddits, and so on. We have choices.

Whether you find your group online or locally, there is support out there for you. That's not to say you won't have to dip your toe in one or more groups before finding the one that's right for you. And if the first one doesn't give you what you're looking for, don't give up!

The Hive weighs in on support groups and why we (mostly) love them:

- definitely not a Lifetime movie -

Carrie • Personally, I didn't want to explore traditional support groups when I was first diagnosed and undergoing treatment. I assumed what they looked and felt like—a bad Lifetime or Hallmark movie. Eventually, I realized I needed to just socialize and be around others who would understand everything I was going through, feeling, and worried about. Only other breast cancer patients can truly relate. Your friends and family can try to be as supportive as possible, but unless they've been through it, they just don't get it.

- *surrogate family* -

Kay • I find my support in our Facebook group and in the women around me. I am truly fortunate to have a village taking ownership in me.

Lavetta • I would like to just say it's best to get in, it's best to join a group. You have to make sure you pick and choose them wisely, because there's a lot of groups that weren't for me; that I wasn't a fit for the group.

- *lifelong friends* -

Carrie • Support groups are so much more than what you see in movies. They're lifelong friendships that form in what could be the toughest period of your life.

Diana • I'm totally in favor of support groups. At first when I was getting a little stronger and I was back home after surgery, I wasn't sure whether or not I wanted to participate in a group. Within two weeks, I met Carrie through a mutual friend. She let me know that Carrie wanted to come over and talk with me; that she was a survivor. Carrie came and stayed for like two hours. We bonded. To me it was very comforting to know that I wasn't alone. I had someone else that understood everything I had gone through.

- the right fit for you -

Lavetta • I was looking for a group of women that were encouraging; that weren't complaining or whining all the time. Groups do things differently, but I needed something different. I needed people that were *alive*. They're going through things like I am, but they still have hope, and they still want to enjoy life.

So yes, by all means, support groups are amazing, if you can find a group that's a fit for you. I found them, and I'm so happy that I did, because I met so many amazing women from all walks of life, all nationalities, that are important to me that have shared and have encouraged me, and I'm thankful for that.

Gina • For me when it comes to a support group, I think you shouldn't jump into it. I think you should definitely take baby steps, and I also think that there's a difference between support and giving someone their opinions as opposed to telling somebody how they should feel. Your story and my story, your cancer and my cancer, your treatment and my treatment are not going to be the same. So when you go to a support group and they're thinking to put you in a category—well, you know what? Your category might not be the same as theirs, and it might not be the right group for you.

T.H. • I had the hardest time with this aspect of my journey. With my initial diagnosis, I felt lost and alone. My mom is a twenty-plus-year breast cancer survivor, but she had a single mastectomy and that was it. No chemo or radiation, and certainly not inflammatory breast cancer. I have friends and neighbors who have been through the trenches, but again, no one who really understood what I was facing.

I tried a couple of online forums dedicated to breast cancer, but they were very cliquish, and I rarely even got a response to my questions, much less a sense of sisterhood. Enter Margaret. I'd read a young adult novel of hers the year before and saw she was promoting a book on life after breast cancer, so I reached out to her. She was genuinely helpful and invited me to an online Facebook group she [and Kayte] created. In that small group, I was the only one with IBC [inflammatory breast cancer] which isn't surprising since it accounts for only about one percent of all breast cancer cases. But I found a community of women who had been through chemo, mastectomy, radiation, and reconstruction. Through that group, I met someone else who knew of an IBC support group, and I joined.

- they really get me! -

Ayanna • Please find a support group that understands your struggles!

Lavetta • The good thing about it is I can share with the sisterhood things that I can't share with my family. I feel like I can't share with them, because they don't really understand. They haven't gone through what I've gone through. The sisterhood, they understand, because they've gone through it. I can just be myself.

Sometimes when you talk about what you've been through, what you're still going through, after everything's been said and done, people get a funny look on their face like they don't want to hear it. When you're in that circle of women—the sisterhood—you can say whatever you want to say, and there's no judgment.

Gina • No matter how much your husband loves you, your mother loves you, your friend loves you, they don't understand. As much as they want to understand and as much as they try to understand, the only people who truly understand are women or men that have been through it. So being part of The CARE Project or being part of any support group of people that have been through what you've been through and are not trying to tell you how to feel is an amazing thing, because they get it. And I think after everything we go through, out of everything that we feel in our hearts, having someone validate our fears, our emotions, our feelings is huge.

Christina • The CARE Project has become my second family, and I do not know what I would have done if I had never been introduced to them by Shannon Kristine Brown. I have found amazing friends/warrior sisters that truly understand what I am going through—whether it is at the beginning of treatment or years out of treatment when everyone thinks we are fine... And we are not.

- I created one -

Bret • Support groups are great. Being able to talk to someone going through the same disease helps you get through it. I didn't have any male support groups, so I didn't have anyone to talk to while I was in treatment. Following treatment, I met others, and we then talked about what we had to go through, and that was reassuring.

I created the Male Breast Cancer Coalition (MBCC) so that no other man would be alone when they hear the words, "You have breast cancer."

- *funny how one thing leads to another* -

Kayte • For me, it all started with Margaret's *Let Me Get This Off My Chest*. Someone sent it to me during one of my last chemotherapies. I was sick in bed, when I heard a knock at the door. I ignored the knock but eventually dragged myself out of bed and found a package with that lovely book inside. I couldn't put it down after I began reading it. It was just what I needed. It made me feel so much less alone. It was so positive and uplifting. Once I finished it, I decided I had to email the author and thank her for her words. She responded, and we have been friends ever since. We decided to start an online support group on Facebook, to help support others, as well.

[*Editor's note: I didn't pay Kayte for this endorsement, but I appreciate it all the same.*]

- *not all rainbows and sunshine* -

T.H. • I've made so many friends in the past three years, in person and online. I've lost a few, too, which never gets easier. As hard as it is to watch someone you know die, I knew I needed to be there for them in the way that I'll need someone if my prognosis ever takes a turn for the worse. A support group is vital to your sanity, but it isn't all rainbows and sunshine; there is a lot of heartache as well.

- *you are not alone* -

Kayte • Being online comes in handy. If you can't sleep and it's

Handle With Care

in the middle of the night, chances are, one of your sisters can't sleep either. Having a group, either in person or online, is so good for your soul. I highly recommend it, even if you're shy and don't want to talk about it much yet. Just reading others' stories will help your heart, like you are a part of a team and not standing alone.

Margaret • Some of us may not have a supportive spouse or close family members. We may already be acting as a caregiver to young children or even taking care of our own parents when we receive our diagnosis (which only adds to the stress of the situation). Receiving a cancer diagnosis can be a very isolating experience as it is. Being part of a support group lets us know we are not alone in our struggles.

- you do you -

S.L. • I'm glad that support groups exist, but they're not for me, and I find it liberating to acknowledge that. Not everyone will respond to cancer and treatment in the same way, and we each need to find the thing that helps us deal. Some people get a ton out of support groups. Personally, what I have found is one-on-one support from friends—ones who share my interests or philosophies but who also have cancer experiences has been the most helpful. I can't thank them enough for answering questions and getting me through.

- voices of experience, mentors -

Margaret • One of the benefits of being part of a support group is that longer-term survivors and thrivers will often act as mentors to those newly diagnosed. They've been there before and are able to provide a shoulder to lean on.

-helped mourn my loss-

Diana • You go through a mourning period, because this is a big part of your body. This is about who you were. Your identification has now been changed, and now you're physically changed. So there's a mourning period that you have to allow yourself to go through, and then, "Okay. Now it's time to move on. Pick yourself up, and let's go." And the gatherings gave me the motivation to do that. It gave me the strength to get out of my house.

Sometimes you go through a depression, and you don't want people to see you. You don't want to see people; you don't want to talk to people. Carrie's invitation to participate at the different events gave me the reason to get out.

- *there is a group for everyone* -

Margaret • Since I've taken part in both online and in-person support groups, I've seen the benefits of each. A local, in-person group can provide a sense of community, of being part of something real. And it certainly gives us the opportunity to dispense plenty of in-person hugs.

Being part of an online community opens up access to those who may live in remote places where there isn't a physical group nearby. Some people don't feel well enough to travel or may not have transportation. An online group can help solve these practical issues while providing needed connection and camaraderie.

Handle With Care

– & –

So what have we learned about support groups?

• Some of us find comfort in groups, online and off, while some of us find comfort in that one friend who's been there.

• We are social animals, and connecting with others going through something similar can be, in itself, a healing experience. So don't be afraid to join a group.

• If you're on the shy side or not able to attend in person, look for a group online.

• You don't have to do this alone.

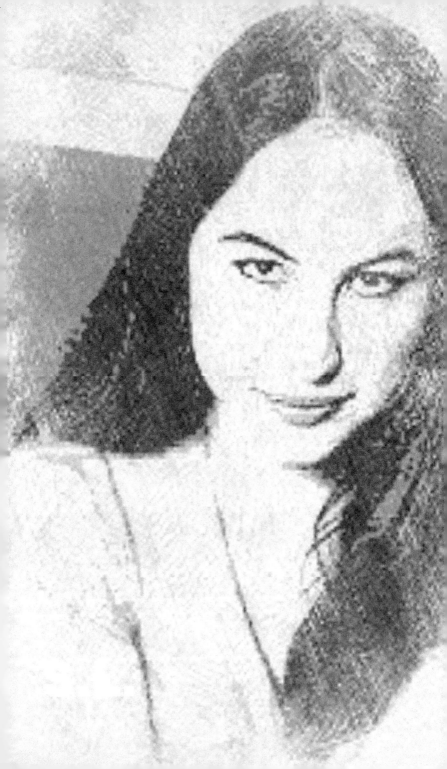

Our Superpower

"Out of suffering have emerged the strongest souls; the most massive characters are seared with scars." ~ Khalil Gibran

Collectively, the Hive has been through a lot. We have overcome long nights; moments when we felt as if we were crumbling on the inside, coming apart, unraveling. Something inside us kept us going until one day we looked back and discovered just how far we've come.

Our strength comes in many forms, often surprising us, teaching us things about ourselves. Somewhere along the way we realized we've gained new powers, or we've tapped into the strength we've had all along.

These are some of our Superpowers:

- *the power of the human body* -

Carrie • Sometimes I look back, and I can't even believe I went through that—being cut hip to hip and armpit to armpit in a fifteen-hour surgery. Pretty horrific. And then almost dying from it. To me, I'm just in awe of our bodies and the ability to heal after such trauma. I can't even call it "my superpower"; I think it's just our body's resilience.

I am in awe of what the human body can withstand. You know, you see these movies with people having chemo, and you see them throwing up and whatever. I didn't have that, but the way I felt, sometimes literally not being able to walk, I can't believe we can go that close to death and come back. Sometimes I go, "Well, you're still here. Pretty freaking crazy." And I look back at all those photos... That's why I took photos along the way, so I can remember and maintain that gratitude just for being here.

- yes, baby steps can be a superpower -

Kayte • My breast cancer absolutely terrified me, at first. I remember getting the news, via a phone call from my OB/GYN, five days after my biopsy. I sobbed like a baby and curled up into a little ball. Eventually I managed to text my sister and have her come over to my house. When she arrived, I passed off my phone to her and told her to be in charge of telling the family. I just lay there in my bed and could hardly breathe. It was like I was grieving my own death but was still alive. A nightmare had just begun and I was so frightened and just wanted to wake up already. My brain wanted, so desperately, to imagine a life after cancer, and to be assured that I would survive. Baby steps are key, though, and they became my superpower.

- superpower? getting through the day -

Kayte • I began focusing on only the day in front of me, and nothing more. I would have an agenda for the day. Show up at such and such appointment. Take my medication at such and

Handle With Care

such time. Pick up my kids from school. Eat dinner. Each time I got something done, it was another check-off on my list of still living my life. It made me feel a sense of accomplishment, even though I had no idea of what was coming next. But each day I survived through was yet another day that made me stronger, more confident, and eventually made my heart heal.

I got through it, one little baby step at a time, and you will, too. So chin up, beautiful.

- *finding the funny* -

Kay • My superpower is the ability to laugh about everything that has happened to me.

Gina • I think I've had my superpower most of my life, and I've tapped into it more because of what we've been through. No matter what you go through, no matter how hard or difficult it may be, you need to (try to) always find a laugh or what makes you happy in between it all. So my superpower is just being a little crazy, a little humorous, and trying to lighten a very harsh moment.

Ayanna • My humor is my superpower. Finding ways and reasons to laugh in your darkest hour is a strength I didn't know I needed until I did.

T.H. • I always assumed I'd fall apart if I ever got cancer. I was a walking train wreck in the weeks leading up to my diagnosis. But once my doctor sat me down and delivered the bad news, a calm settled over me, and somehow, I didn't freak out. Over the next year, I learned that I have the ability to find humor in nearly every situation, and that humor kept me going through some of my darkest days. Laughing my way through treatment and recovery was cathartic in a way I never anticipated.

- *sheer strength* -

Lavetta • The only thing that comes to mind is the strength to keep going, to live, to keep moving. I'm fifty-five. I never would have thought at age twenty-five that I ever would have gone through what I'm going through with my body. If only I could tell myself at twenty-five, "You're going to be okay, Lavetta. You're going to be strong at fifty-five." I've got the strength of being strong.

Christina • My superpower: The ability to overcome anything that comes at me, because if I defeated CANCER, I can overcome and defeat anything else.

- *we persevere* -

Lavetta • Perservering through everything. Sometimes I even come to question myself. It's like during the whole ordeal that I was going through, I knew that I was going to be okay. I still believe I'm going to be okay. Through the chemo, through the surgery, I never doubted that I was not going to be okay.

I ask myself, "Are you okay? You're not down and out? You're not destroyed by this?" And I went to my pastor, and I was like,

Handle With Care

"Should I be acting this way? I'm just okay."

He said, "That's the way you're supposed to be, Lavetta, because you have the Lord on your side, and he's given you that strength to go through this."

- *open book* -

Margaret • This might sound strange, but "vulnerability" popped into my mind. Being confronted with my mortality made me want to share something real with people, even if it meant exposing myself to possible ridicule. I wanted to delve deeper into my emotions, sharing my fears, the funny stuff, the impact breast cancer has made on my life, even how it's affected me professionally. So vulnerability is definitely one of my unexpected new superpowers.

- *I'll keep on tomorrow, too* -

S.L. • It's not easy, afterward. I didn't get better and then move on the way I wanted to. I didn't pick myself up and dust off my knees. My career got derailed, my savings got used up, my life went in a totally different direction. Nothing made me stronger— it just sucked.

But—I'm still here. I'm still going. I found a new career. I still lose it over long-reaching effects of the cancer that affect my life today, and it still broke things inside of me that aren't fixed yet. But I'm still here. There's a strength to me in acknowledging all this. That some of us do break, some of us aren't endlessly "strong," and we can't always pick up all the pieces before they get stepped on or kicked under the couch. And it's... Okay, if that's us. We're not lesser or deficient because we can't snap back from trauma as readily as another person. Because our healing curve is longer and might never be without cracks. Keeping on after doesn't have to look like a victory to be important. I'll keep on tomorrow, too—that's the strength I've got, the one I didn't know I'd need.

- *reclaiming our time* -

Margaret • I'm definitely pickier with how I use my time now, so I guess another superpower is not putting up with things. You won't find me waiting in line for hours to try the hot new theme park ride when I could be sitting in the shade, sipping on a mocha, checking out the appetizer menu. Or (even better) maybe taking a rest on one of those coin-operated foot massagers.

- *patience and perspective* -

Diana • It's a double-edged sword. In some instances there are things that I won't put up with anymore because of the fact that I've learned that I have to live life to the fullest every day. I was given an opportunity to live; therefore, I can't waste it.

On the other hand, it has given me more patience. And I had patience before, but not like this. With some things.

With other things, I have no patience whatsoever.

So patience and compassion where I didn't have them before,

Handle With Care

and that is a big learning lesson. Before I would make a big thing out of nothing, and now? No. No.

I think patience is my thing.

But... Like I said, there are other things that are not a priority, and it pisses me off, and I say, "Oh, hell, no. I'm not going to do that."

It's given me perspective.

I think that's my superpower. Perspective.

So what have we learned about our Superpowers?

• We are strong (even though we may have felt pushed to our absolute physical limits).

• We've been through it, each of us, one foot ahead of the other, and you will, too.

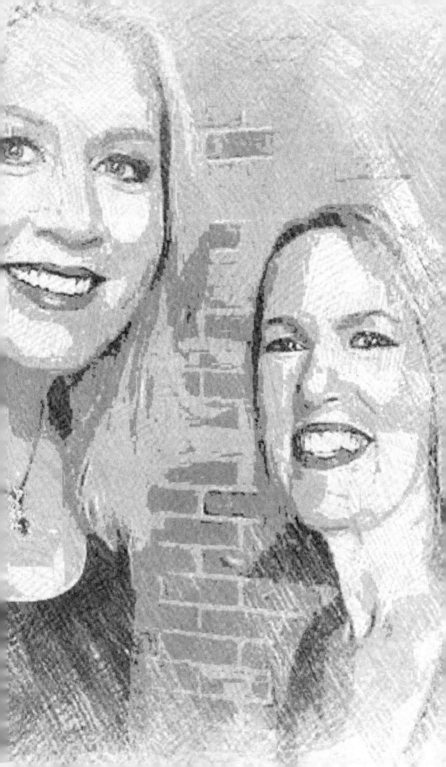

What We Are Thankful For

While it may seem counter-intuitive to talk about things for which we are thankful while dealing with the wretchedness of a cancer diagnosis, giving thanks shifts us from a perspective of "Why me?" to "I have so much. How am I so fortunate?" When we act from a space of gratitude, we possess the ability to turn our negative emotions upside down. And our "thank you's" don't have to be big things, they can be little things such as having rides to our appointments, or the friend who simply sits with us, listens, and makes us laugh. Our spouse, our kids, our dog, our cat, our coffee, our dark chocolate, the ocean, our lip gloss...

Here are a few things for which the Hive gives thanks:

- I'm still here -

Carrie • I'm thankful to still be here eight years out. I still think about recurrence every single day. So I'm thankful to be here.

- our personal village -

Kay • Perspective and resources: This includes family, friends and work.

I'm happy to have everything structural and emotional that I need to help me in my journey of managing this disease.

Also, I'm thankful for my orientation as a person. Practicality, and a sense of purpose has helped.

T.H. • I have so much to be thankful for. I had an incredible support system during treatment, including my immediate family —my sisters who drove me to and from appointments, my new sister-in-law who took me to the hospital for reconstruction surgery when my husband was out of town so I wouldn't have to Uber, and my neighbors who organized meals so we didn't have to worry about cooking during treatment.

Diana • I am grateful for the people that I have met, for the doctors who were so wonderful, and the staff.

I'm grateful for waking up every day and taking on whatever today brings my way.

I am grateful for all of my friends who supported me during this time, because I had a great group of friends who took me for my treatments and took me for my radiation. My best friend coordinated everyone, so one week, two or three of them would be responsible for me that week, and then the next week somebody else. They took time out of their lives to help me.

- *our health and connections* -

T.H. • I'm beyond blessed at having a pathological complete response to chemo, upping my odds for survival and significantly reducing my chance of developing lymphedema.

Handle With Care

I'm grateful for the amazing friends I've made on this journey, at chemo and through online and in-person support groups. We may only have one thing in common, "breast cancer," but sometimes that's all it takes to bond on a deeper level. Finding people who really understand chemo brain, phantom pain, and the fact that aches and pains or a weird rash can no longer just be ignored, helps ground me on a daily basis.

Christina • I am thankful for all the love I have found through my diagnosis and for the strength I feel I developed through my journey. I have met so many beautiful souls—survivors and non-survivors—after my diagnosis.

Carrie • I'm thankful to have lived long enough to be a grandmother.

Lavetta • I am just so thankful that I am still here. I was cancer-free for one year, and in 2018, I had a recurrence, and I come to find out it's Stage IV, metastatic to my bones. There's no cure for that, it's just stay on maintenance drugs, if that's what you decide to do. But I am thankful, through everything that I've been through, that I'm still here walking around. I can see, feel, and touch; that I'm still alive. Some of my friends that were diagnosed before me and even after me, some of them are not here.

Kayte • SO THANKFUL for my health. I will never take it for granted, again. So thankful to be six years cancer-free, and that I've been blessed with getting to watch my boys grow up into adulthood (for the most part, at least. They are nineteen and seventeen now).

So thankful for the rest of my family, and all of my friends who have stood by my side throughout this roller coaster of a journey.

And last, but certainly not least, SO THANKFUL for all the new friends I've gained along the way, my new sisters. They understood me like no one else could. I wasn't alone in my fight and never will be. I know they will be my friends for life, and we have an emotional bond that cannot be broken.

- *medical care providers* -

Margaret • One thing in particular I give thanks for—a very big thing—is the medical care I have received. From the time my cancer was caught at the age of thirty-four to my recurrence twelve years later, my medical team has given me top-notch care and continue to follow me to this day.

I am thankful for medical professionals working in the field, as well as the researchers who dedicate their lives to coming up with cures and life-saving treatments for not only cancer, but other diseases and life-changing conditions.

- *new friends* -

Carrie • I am most thankful for finding the friends that I have now through breast cancer. The people that I know now—I should say the people that surround me now—I only know because of breast cancer. Almost every single one of them. I'm so thankful for those people, because I know they'll be there till the end of my life.

Probably second is the people that I've met.

Handle With Care

Third is finding the purpose for the last half of my life, which is The CARE Project and helping others get through it.

- *my people* -

S.L. • The people. I am one hundred percent thankful for the people in my life. I had incredible support. Caretaking, patient advocacy, insurance and unemployment logistics, emotional bulwarking. They covered exactly what I needed done and backed off where I told them that "help" was actually unhelpful, which is one of the greatest gifts of all.

Ayanna • I'm thankful to God for helping me get through this.

I'm thankful for the love and support from my family.

And I'm thankful for Carrie Madrid and The CARE Project, Inc. for the support of the ladies who went through it and are going through it.

Bret • I am thankful for family and friends. Without them, going through cancer would be impossible.

Gina • My support group was amazing. I have a big family—I'm the youngest of five. One of my most memorable times, I had just lost my hair, and the vanity of it all was just something I could not believe. I was a tomboy; I wasn't one of those prissy girls. So it's really funny. I didn't think the vanity part of losing my breasts and losing my hair would be so big for me, but it was.

I was going into my worst days in my second round of chemo,

I'd lost my hair, so I was feeling pretty low. And I don't do that very often, it was just one of those moments. My sister called me and asked me how I was doing, and I was kind of pouty and not feeling very well and just kind of telling her about my hair. So my "fam bam" called each other without me knowing. They called my son and told him to leave the front door open and that they were going to come over.

Well, they all met up, and the door opens, and they've got music going, and they're coming in dancing and singing to me and just lifting me up. It was amazing. It was such a beautiful moment.

So what have we learned about being thankful?

• There is nothing like going through a harrowing, potentially life-threatening experience to cause us to evaluate and re-order our lives.

• We have the potential to embrace thankfulness even on our worst days.

• Giving thanks gives us power.

• We have so much to be thankful for.

Handle With Care

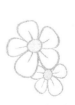

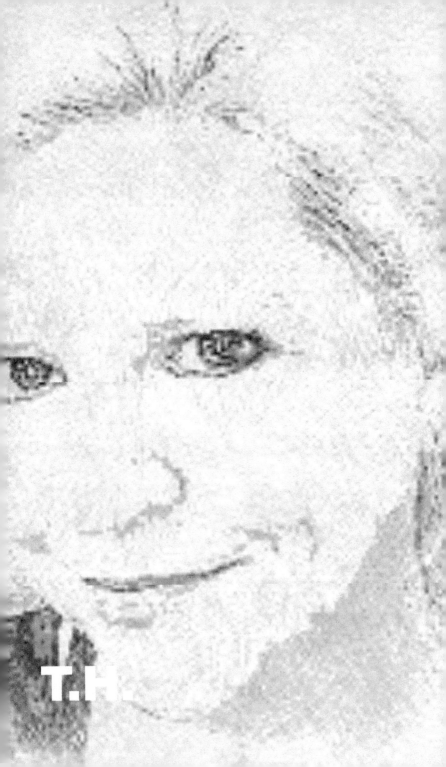
T.H.

Epiphanies, Life Lessons, and Moving Forward

It's a stretch of the imagination to think that a person can go through the whole range of emotions that accompany a breast cancer diagnosis, treatment, then life afterwards without picking up a little insight along the way. We might experience that "Aha!" moment while sitting in our oncologist's waiting room, or during those impossible nights when we're fighting for sleep as competing thoughts and fears run wild through our minds.

We learn, whether we planned it that way or not, because that is how life is.

From the spectacular to the ordinary, here are a few of the things we've learned:

- old sayings hang around for a reason -

Carrie • As for a life lesson, you know all those old cliches that we've heard our entire lives? "Life is too short"; "Don't sweat the small stuff"; "It's just a blip on the radar in the grand scheme of things"? All of those sayings that we get super annoyed that our parents or whoever told us? Well, it turns out it's all true.

Kay • Life is also in the small, annoying moments, not just the grand and touching.

T.H. • I don't know that I ever had an epiphany in the true sense of the word. I had little moments when I'd remind myself that life is short, precious, and not to be wasted, rather than one big 'Aha' moment. Over time, I learned that a breast is just a breast. I don't need it to function in my daily life, and it doesn't define me in the way I once thought it did. I realized that life is lived in the here and now, but that doesn't mean I can't plan for a future. I came to accept that my life will never be the way it was before, and that I'm surprisingly okay with that.

Christina • I think that for me it is beginning to understand why some of our fighters earn their wings and some of us survive to care for others.

Carrie • We're given this term "breast cancer survivor," and I'm proud to say that. And I know not everybody likes the term; there's a lot of verbiage around that. But while I'm technically a breast cancer survivor, I'm really living life now, and I was just surviving before breast cancer. I was surviving mentally, emotionally, physically as a single mom. Financially, I was just surviving. Now, even though I don't have a lot of money, I feel like I'm really living.

- *silver linings* -

Margaret • For me it was more a gradual awakening, a clarity that I don't think I had before, where I evaluated my life and realized that the important things were the people closest to me. The feelings I had for my family and friends deepened as the acquisition of material goods and the pursuit of wealth faded into the background.

T.H. • Until you go through it, it's hard to explain, but ask any cancer survivor and they will likely tell you that there are big silver linings to be found in all the ugly storm clouds. You learn to appreciate life and health and everyday moments in a way that was impossible before. Living through cancer is transformational on a very basic level, and yet I'm still the same me I've always been, but with a few more scars, and a whole new load of attitude!

- *living in the moment* -

Lavetta • My thing for me right now, even during the time I was going through treatment—you know, you spend a lot of time by yourself—I know I did when I was going through treatment. My big thing is: Live in the moment. Take each day, one day at a time. Just live in the moment, because you don't know what tomorrow is going to bring, and yesterday is gone.

Before, I was the type of person, you know, a planner. It was always, "I have to take care of this tomorrow," you know, "I don't know if I did that yesterday," using up today thinking about yesterday and tomorrow. That was a big, big thing for me.

- *cool your jets* -

Gina • For me, I think the biggest life lesson is: You need to slow down. You need to slow down, and you need to not stress so much. I definitely was very high strung, and just being that high-strung person that I was, I wasn't helping myself.

My epiphany is just: You can't take care of anybody else until you take care of yourself first.

- *relationships become defined* -

Kayte • Relationships are the first thing that came to mind when I thought about epiphanies and life lessons that my breast cancer has given to me. I like to think of my breast cancer as a filter. It captured all my true friends, and held onto them tight, while all the others slipped right on through.

At first I was shocked by losing any. I assumed that everyone would be right by my side. But some people just can't hang. They were obviously in my life at the time because it was convenient, I was fun to be around, et cetera. But as soon as times got tough, they were nowhere to be found. Yet, others, I saw even more after my diagnosis. Some, who I didn't think were that close to me before, and more like acquaintances, majorly stepped up and continued to feed me, listen to me vent, make me smoothies, and anything else they could possibly think of in an effort of making me feel better and showing me their love.

Handle With Care

• One thing the Hive has collectively learned from our experiences: Life really is short, so let's not waste our precious time by fighting with people over petty things. Let us love those around us, taking joy in the small things, appreciating our lives and each other.

• Laugh, enjoy that plate of tacos, pet the dog, love those you love, and don't forget: Turn the music up loud once in a while and really move.

• Dance like no one is watching.

• Thank you for spending this time with us, and remember to take a moment to look up to the skies once in a while. When you need support, look to one of the many of us who have walked this road. And we are everywhere.

• You are not alone.

• Oh, and one last thing..!

Don't forget to laugh.
And don't forget your lip gloss.

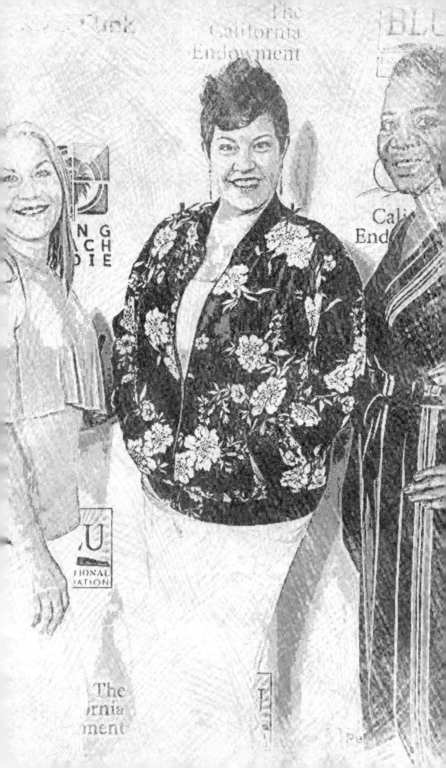

The Hive's Bios

Carrie Madrid is the co-founder of **The CARE Project, Inc**. In 2017, she was honored as one of the Latinas of Influence at Hispanic Lifestyle's 2017 Latina Conference. She dedicates her life to helping others, raising public awareness of male and female breast cancer, and has been featured keynote speaker for events sponsored by UC Riverside, Kaiser Foundation, and many other organizations. She probably enjoys calamari more than most and makes it a point to never miss a UCR home basketball game.

Margaret Lesh is the author of **Let Me Get This Off My Chest: A Breast Cancer Survivor Over-Shares**, as well as several other books and short stories. She is currently working on a slightly tragic love story but promises it will have a happy-ish ending. She runs on tacos, human kindness, The Beatles, and the occasional gin & tonic. To learn more about her books, visit her website margaretlesh.com.

T.H. Hernandez is the author of young adult novels *The Union* and *Superhero High*, among others. She thrives on coffee, pumpkin-flavored anything, Doctor Who marathons, Bad Lip Reading videos, and all things young adult (especially the three young adults who share her home). Diagnosed with inflammatory breast cancer in 2016, she appreciates every day life has given her since then. She has been disease free for nearly three years. Follow her on Twitter at @TheresaHernandz

S.L. Huang writes books, mostly about angry women who shoot at people. She's had cancer twice now (because she's just that thorough). Her short science fiction allegory about her experience with breast cancer was republished in The *Best American Science Fiction and Fantasy 2016* and longlisted for the BSFA Award. You can buy her books or follow her online at slhuang.com or on Twitter at @sl_huang.

Kayte Faulconer is an RN case manager dedicated to helping others, especially mentoring those working through their own breast cancer diagnoses. With seemingly endless energy and optimism, Kayte tries her best to make the world a better place. (If we could only bottle her energy, we'd be able to power the globe.) Check out her website, ketokayte.com to learn about all things related to the ketogenic diet.

Kay Hsu is Global Director of Instagram Creative Shop, as well as being an all-around phenomenal person who makes everyone within her orbit feel energized and better for knowing her. A passionate fundraising advocate, she's raised an incredible amount of money for **CancerCare**, a nonprofit dedicated to providing free counseling and support services for anyone affected by cancer.

Gina Negrete Fitzsimmons works for Toyota Corporation and has literally never met a stranger. She's famous for her group selfies, her love of life, her giving nature, and mentoring others going through breast cancer. She's often asked to speak about her experiences with breast cancer, and is also a passionate advocate for Type 1 Diabetes research, education and awareness. She loves all things '80s.

Lavetta Ross is in graduate school, studying to become a marriage and family therapist. Though she leads a hectic life between work and school, to be around Lavetta is to feel as if you're in the presence of someone who has everything figured out. She has a beautiful smile and enjoys living life to the fullest. She is not one to pass up a dance floor.

Diana Jaurigue is the consummate office manager who will whip your place into shape in no time. But the really important thing about Diana: She gives the world's best hugs, and you're happier just being around her. She's a kind, caring mentor to breast cancer patients and a vital part of The CARE Project as well as an avid gardener. She runs with a large squad of long-time friends (and tries her best to stay out of trouble).

Christina Villanueva is a two-time survivor and works for Concentra Health and is a dedicated member of The CARE Project, devoted to helping and mentoring others. Beautiful inside and out, Christina enjoys traveling to Guanajuato, Mexico, and spending time with those she loves. (She also enjoys the occasional Margarita.)

Ayanna Clark works in customer service, and is a talented artist with a passion for writing. If she seems quiet, it's probably because she's studying the scene, trying to figure out how she's going to turn you into a cartoon. She's a firm believer that pineapple, in fact, does belong on pizza. Check her art out on RedBubble redbubble.com/people/navayaart

Bret Miller is the co-founder of **Male Breast Cancer Coalition**, a group he began in 2013 with the help of his parents (Director) Peggy and Bob, brother Blake, and co-founder Cheri Ambrose. Bret is dedicated to spreading the word about male breast cancer and being an advocate for other men dealing with male breast cancer. Plus, he's a really good guy.

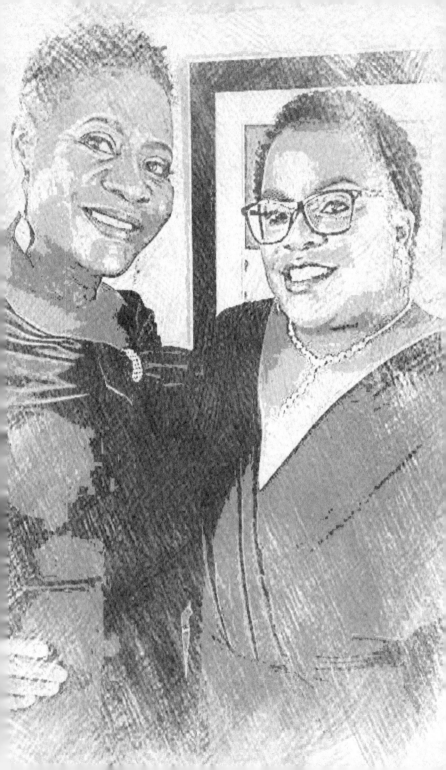

My Favorite Quote

"Your life is your story. Write well. Edit often." ~ Susan Statham

As has been said so often, words matter, so we're closing by sharing words that inspired us, gave us strength, resonated with us in some way, maybe even made us laugh out loud.

Here are a few of our favorites:

Carrie • I read a quote years ago, and it stuck with me. And my kids, when they ask me for a quote for anything, I always tell them, "Pain is inevitable, but misery is an option."

I live my life by that, and it just rolled into cancer as well. Pain was inevitable, in that I was going to have surgery and chemo and all that—radiation, and open wounds, and surgery after surgery— but I didn't have to be miserable. Perspective is everything.

Christina • There is a post I saw on Facebook that I really loved and feel that it confirmed my want and thirst to live my life as if it is the last day. It was a cartoon of a conversation that Charlie Brown is having with Snoopy. Charlie Brown tells Snoopy, "We only live once, Snoopy," and Snoopy replies back, "Wrong! We only die once. We live every day."

Lavetta • Matthew 6:33. "But seek first the kingdom of God and His righteousness, and all these things will be added unto you."

Gina • For me it's always been Scripture. I know there are all these quotes about being strong—and all of that is so true—but for me what I always tell myself over and over again: "Thy will be done."

And, of course, "Don't Stop Believin'."

[*Journey fans in the Hive.*]

Bret • My favorite quote is from the movie Van Wilder. (I am sure it was said by someone more famous, but it really stuck with me.)

"Don't take life too seriously. You'll never get out alive."

Cancer is a serious diagnosis, it is a life-or-death situation, but if all you think about is death and don't start to live your life to the fullest, it *will* be the end. Enjoy life, have fun, make jokes—because in the end, we only have one life to live.

Margaret • I have two...

"You are not as important as you think."

I love this quote because it's a reminder that the thing I'm obsessing about, I can probably ratchet the stress level down a few notches. Not everything is the end of the world. It's a good perspective check. Plus, it makes me laugh.

One of the most beautiful quotes I've come across is from Emily Dickinson's poem, "Hope is the Thing with Feathers." When we're going through hard times, if we have a kernel of hope

Handle With Care

that we will get through the next minute or the next hour or the next day, then we have something to hold onto. Hope urges us to hang on a little while longer; things will get better...

Hope is the thing with feathers

That perches in the soul

And sings the tune without the words

And never stops at all

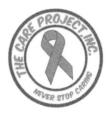

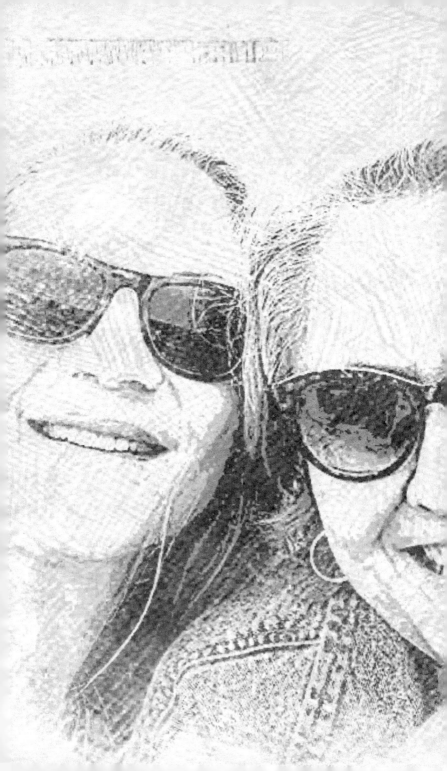

- *trust your gut* -

Ayanna • You have to trust your body, even when you don't want to believe what it's telling you.

- *you realize who your friends are* -

Kayte • I think tragedy has a way of filtering the true friends from the not so true. So now I cherish those true friendships that much more. They are my forever friends who aren't going anywhere, no matter what.

- *epiphanies? hah!* -

S.L. • Epiphanies? None. Well, one: Cancer sucks.

- *it's okay to need a little help* -

Diana • I went from completely independent and in control to releasing and letting everyone else take over. It was really a big step for me.

- *loving my (new) self* -

Carrie • I learned how to truly love and appreciate myself from the inside out. Growing up, I had too-large breasts, and long, thick hair, and everybody knew me as "the girl with the big hair and the big boobs." Losing that, for me, wasn't a devastating thing, it was more like an "Oh, thank God, I can get rid of them. I have an excuse."

It was very liberating. I really felt like I was stripped down and re-born in terms of my body. People may find it hard to believe, but I, honest, to goodness, mean this. Eight years ago, when I was forty years old and going in for that first mammogram after I found my lump, I was more aesthetically pleasing according to society—face, body, skin, teeth, everything —and afterwards, I am weathered. But I will say that while I looked pretty good for forty, now I look at myself, and I'm like, "You are a badass." I know that I am a much more beautiful spirit and soul than I was when I "looked" better.

So what we have learned about those epiphanies, life lessons, and moving on?

• We know there aren't many certainties in life (other than the old saying about death and taxes; right? You've heard that one before). Life is life. We encounter challenges and roadblocks. We face them; we go around them; we move ahead.

Handle With Care

48302615R00084